Frontiers of Medicine

Frontiers of Medicine

Foundations for the Future

TORSTAR BOOKS
New York • Toronto

TORSTAR BOOKS INC.
41 Madison Avenue, Suite 2900
New York, NY 10010

THE HUMAN BODY
Frontiers of Medicine:
Foundations for the Future

Publisher
Bruce Marshall

Art Editor
John Bigg

Creation Coordinator
Harold Bull

Editor
John Clark

Managing Editor
Ruth Binney

Commissioning Editor
Hal Robinson

Contributors
Arthur Boylston, Julian Chomet, Colin Fergusson, Peter Howell, Steve Parker, Saffron Whitehead

Text Editors
Wendy Allen, Mike Darton, James McCarter, Maria Pal

Researchers
Angela Bone, Jazz Wilson

Picture Researchers
Jan Croot, Dee Robinson

Layout and Visualization
Rita Wuthrich

Artists
Mick Gillah, Mick Saunders, Rob Shone, Shirley Willis

Cover Design
Moonink Communications

Cover Art
Paul Giovanopoulos

Production Director
Barry Baker

Production Coordinator
Janice Storr

Business Coordinator
Candy Lee

Planning Assistant
Avril Essery

International Sales
Barbara Anderson

RA
418.5
.M4
F76
1986

In conjunction with this series Torstar Books offers an electronic digital thermometer which provides accurate body temperature readings in large liquid crystal numbers within 60 seconds.

For more information write to:
Torstar Books Inc.
41 Madison Avenue, Suite 2900
New York, NY 10010

Marshall Editions, an editorial group that specializes in the design and publication of scientific subjects for the general reader, prepared this book. Marshall has written and illustrated standard works on technology, animal behavior, computer usage and the tropical rain forests which are recommended for schools and libraries as well as for popular reference.

Series Consultants

Donald M. Engelman is Professor of Molecular Biophysics and Biochemistry and Professor of Biology at Yale. He has pioneered new methods for understanding cell membranes and ribosomes, and has also worked on the problem of atherosclerosis. He has published widely in professional and lay journals and lectured at many universities and international conferences. He is also involved with National Advisory Groups concerned with Molecular Biology, Cancer, and the operation of National Laboratory Facilities.

Harold C. Slavkin, Professor of Biochemistry at the University of Southern California, directs the Graduate Program in Craniofacial Biology and also serves as Chief of the Laboratory for Developmental Biology in the University's Gerontology Center. His research on the genetic basis of congenital defects of the head and neck has been widely published.

Lewis Thomas is Chancellor of the Memorial Sloan-Kettering Cancer Center in New York City and University Professor at the State University of New York, Stony Brook. A member of the National Academy of Sciences, Dr. Thomas has served on advisory councils of the National Institutes of Health.

Consultants for Frontiers of Medicine

Murray Eden is Chief of Biomedical Engineering and Instrumentation Branch, National Institutes of Health. He is also Professor of Electrical Engineering (Emeritus) at the Massachusetts Institute of Technology. He has been lecturer in the Department of Preventive Medicine, Harvard Medical School and visiting professor at the Johns Hopkins University and the Swiss Federal Polytechnic Institute at Lausanne. He is coauthor of *Engineering and Living Systems* and coeditor of *Recognizing Patterns, Microcomputers in Patient Care* and *Contemporary Biomaterials.* He is also the author or coauthor of more than one hundred articles concerned with health research instrumentation, mathematical models in biology, image processing and pattern recognition.

Stanley Joel Reiser is Griff T. Ross Professor of Humanities and Technology in Health Care at the University of Texas Health Science Center in Houston. He is the author of *Medicine and the Reign of Technology,* coeditor of *Ethics in Medicine: Historical Perspectives and Contemporary Concerns,* and of *The Machine at the Bedside: Strategies for Using Technology in Patient Care,* and coeditor of the anthology *The Machine at the Bedside.*

Medical Advisor

Arthur Boylston

**Library of Congress
Cataloging in Publication Data**

Main entry under title:

Frontiers of Medicine

Includes index.
1. Medical innovations. 2. Medicine.
1. Title. [DNLM: 1. Medicine—trends—popular works.   WB 130 F935]
RA418.5.M4F76 1986   610   86–1368
ISBN 0-920269-95-8

ISBN 0-920269-22-2 (The Human Body series)
ISBN 0-920269-95-8 (Frontiers of Medicine)
ISBN 1-55001-004-2 (leatherbound)
ISBN 0-920269-97-4 (school ed.)

20 19 18 17 16 15 14 13 12 11
10   9   8   7   6   5   4   3   2   1

Printed in Belgium

Contents

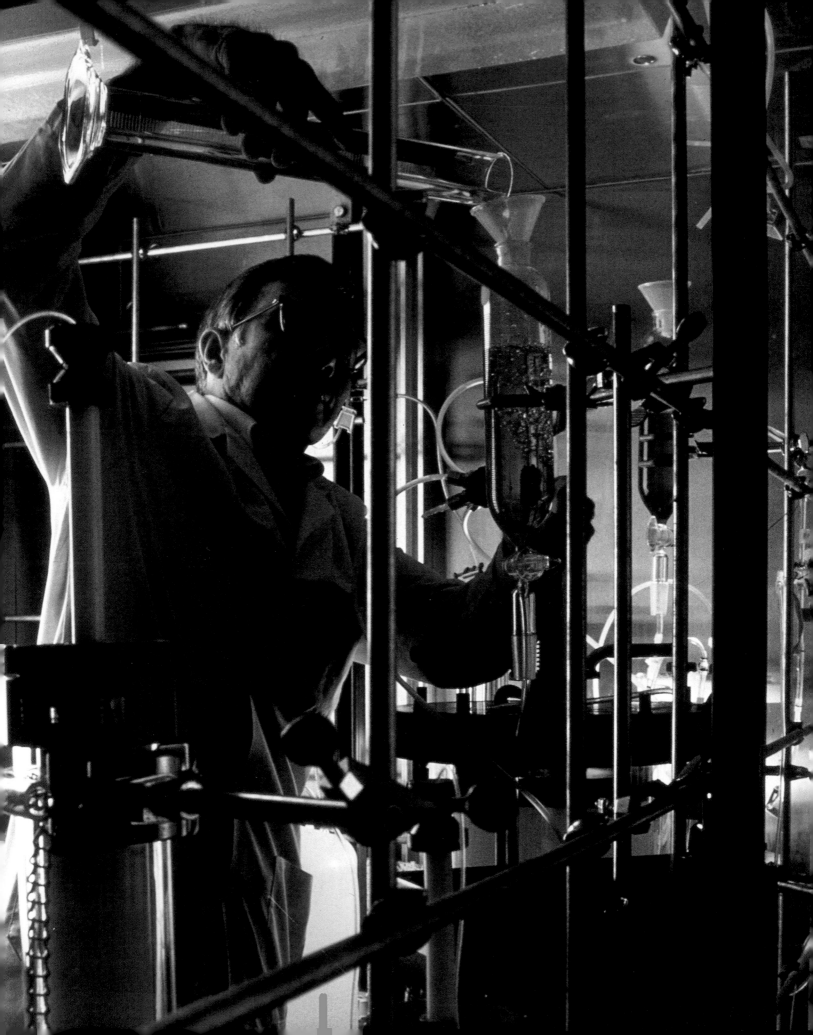

Introduction:

Toward a Healthier World

Never before have laboratory scientists made such major contributions to medicine. In the area of chemotherapy, researchers continue the search for new drugs and other biologically active substances, and for ways of extracting or synthesizing them. In molecular biology, scientists probe the innermost secrets of the cell, analyzing the composition and structure of proteins, nucleic acids and even genes, which ultimately control all the biological activity of the human body.

Who would have believed, a century ago, that by the mid-1980s scientists would have solved many of the serious medical problems that then plagued the populations of the world, only to be faced with new difficulties?

The question may in itself seem rather pessimistic, even daunting. But that is to overlook the fact that a century ago physicians were already considerably in advance of the physicians of a century earlier, and *they* were far ahead of medical experts even earlier — and so on back.

Present-day medicine thus owes much to the discoveries and techniques of the past. Yet the rate at which progress is now being made, at which new discoveries follow one another, and at which new techniques, new pieces of equipment — even whole new fields of study — are being devised, is prodigiously fast, and still accelerating.

The results are plain to see. Today's hospitals can boast of transplant and replacement surgery, laser techniques, microsurgery, and the fitting of computerized prosthetics. Computer-controlled scanning methods permit accurate diagnosis of disorders that affect internal body structures. Local physicians are able to prescribe from a wealth of beneficial drugs, and to use any of a number of forms of treatment, all guaranteed to help those in need. Research into disease and suffering of all kinds continues urgently, and with increasing success. Much of the entire world has been educated to think in terms of its health. Even commerce is taking advantage of the innovations afforded by genetic engineering. These great capabilities were, until recently, all in the realm of the fantastic.

What frontiers still remain to be crossed? Can today's rate of advance in medical experience be sustained? It is possible, through these pages, to look ahead a little. What can be seen there gives grounds for optimism. Caution must remain the watchword, but the overall picture of the future remains one of humankind hopeful of a healthier, happier way of life.

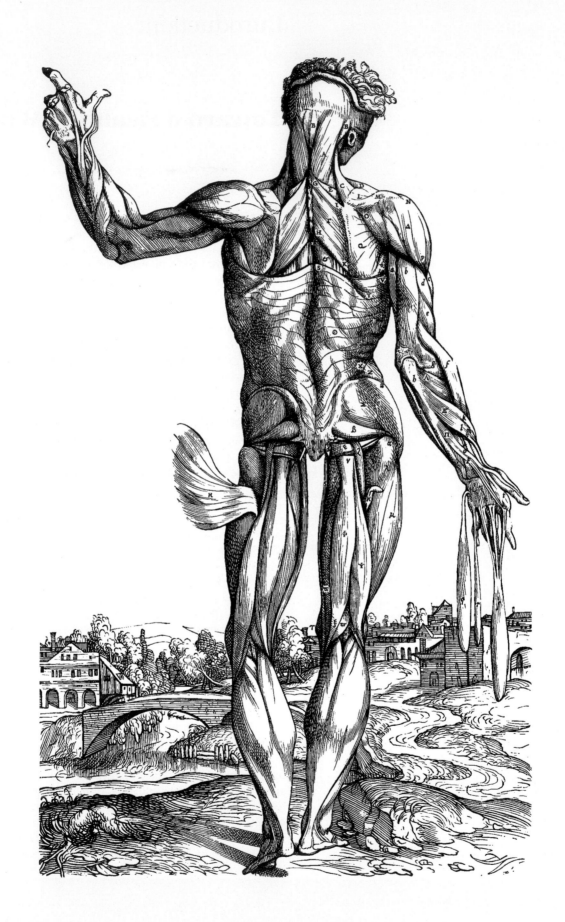

Chapter 1

Progress of Medicine

The future of medicine and the future of humankind will inevitably be intertwined. With an ever-expanding world population — even assuming that technological advances will provide enough food and shelter for everyone — the burden of maintaining a meaningful quality of life increasingly will be carried on the shoulders of the medical profession.

A brief account of the history and development of this most human of the sciences is vital to any reasoned projection into the future of medicine. It is a story of accelerating insight and achievement, but at the same time a story of occasional intransigence and bigotry in the face of what today would be regarded as incontrovertible evidence.

In modern times, medicine has brought together the initially disparate disciplines of biology and chemistry, given additional credibility to psychology, and demonstrated the fundamental significance of genetics and molecular biology. Despite the historical reluctance of medical science to assimilate the benefits of other domains of scholarship, modern medicine has been able to draw avidly on all sorts of expertise — from atomic physics to computer science — in order to increase its effectiveness.

If the foundation of medicine is a conscious attempt by mankind to fight disease, then medicine surely must be as old as human consciousness. Little is known about its origins. For primitive mankind medicine was probably based on herbal magic and ritual practices. In the great early civilizations simple theories of health and disease were formulated which led to a more systematic approach toward medicine, although for thousands of years medicine remained inextricably linked with demons, gods, evil spirits and sorcery.

The system of medicine begun by the Sumerians more than five thousand years ago, which was adopted by the Babylonians of Mesopotamia and later by the Egyptians, was connected to, and influenced by, cosmic phenomena corresponding

Medicine developed from myth and magic into a rational, healing science only after a detailed knowledge of the anatomy of the human body became available. Often, taboo and religious observances prohibited dissection of corpses. This illustration is from Vesalius' De humani corporis fabrica, *published in 1543. A monumental and beautiful work, based on acute experimental observation rather than on dogma, it overturned many previously accepted ideas about the structure of the human body.*

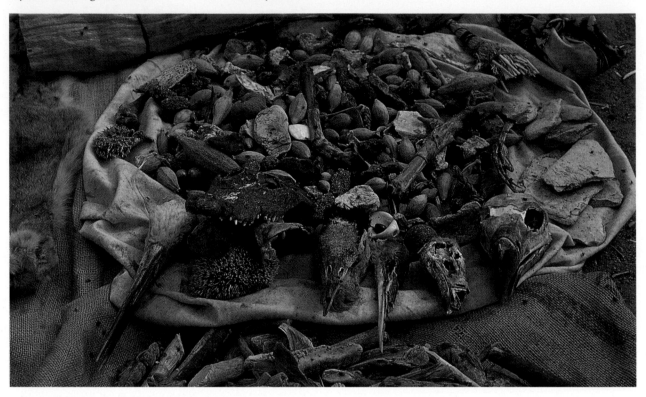

to the condition of the universe. Any disease or disorder had first to be categorized with the aid of religion, magic, natural lore and science.

The ancient Chinese emperors of about three thousand years ago adopted a system of treatments that were based on the idea of two opposing principles: the Yang and the Yin. The Yang principle was positive, active and masculine, as signified by the sky, light, strength, hardness, warmth and dryness. The Yin principle was negative, passive and feminine, and was signified by the moon, earth, darkness, weakness, cold and moisture.

The practice of acupuncture evolved from the ideas of Yin and Yang. By inserting needles accurately into strategic points of the body, it was thought that any imbalance between Yang and Yin could be redressed. In their medicine, therefore, the Chinese sought to cure the symptoms of disease by reestablishing an internal harmony.

The Chinese were also great herbalists, as the writings ascribed to the legendary emperor Shen Nung reveal. *Pen T'sao Ching*, or *The Great Herbal*, written nearly 5,000 years ago, lists 365 herbs,

prescriptions and potions, including some of today's familiar drugs. Opium, for example, is described as a painkiller, rhubarb as a laxative, and kaolin is recommended for diarrhea.

Hellenic Schools of Healing

In the ancient Greek civilizations from about 1000 B.C., medicine was strongly influenced by the belief in numerous deities who were able to cure or to prevent disease. This is particularly well represented by the cult of Asklepios, or Aesculapius. A number of magnificent temples were built in his name, usually on sites with commanding views over the Mediterranean Sea.

In these temples, which became sanctuaries of healing, priests ministered to the sick and charged fees according to the patient's ability to pay. Although this cult lasted for more than ten centuries — and well into the Christian era — many became skeptical of the mystical element in healing, and lay medicine became popular.

The medical school that is best documented was on the Greek island of Cos where Hippocrates, one

Opium, extracted from the juice of unripe seed-heads of poppies (below left), is one of mankind's oldest drugs; it appears in ancient Assyrian medical texts dating from almost three thousand years ago. Even today, as its derivative morphine, it is the physician's mainstay in the relief of severe pain, particularly in the treatment of cancer patients. Modern chemotherapy to treat cancer often requires the administration of a combination of drugs known as a "cocktail", prepared (below right) in a sterile cabinet. The mixture includes a painkiller as well as drugs that specifically attack the cancerous cells in the body.

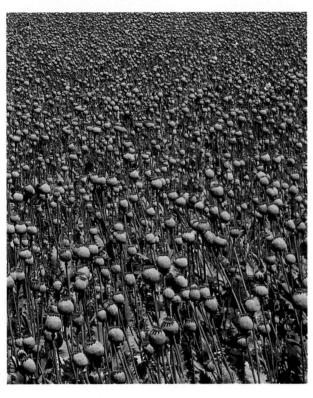
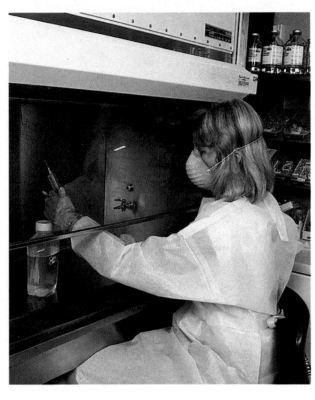

of the greatest figures in the history of medicine, lived and worked. Born around 460 B.C., Hippocrates was respected not only as a great physician but also as an inspired teacher. The famous Oath attributed to him represents the basic code of ethics to be followed by medical practitioners, and its principles are still adhered to by physicians today. His system of diagnosis, based on acute observation and reason, established the foundations of medical practice for centuries.

The weakness of Hippocratic medicine resulted from only a primitive knowledge of anatomy and physiology. At that time the body was considered to contain four humors — black bile, yellow bile, blood and phlegm — associated with the four elements of earth, fire, air and water. Disease was thought to be caused by an imbalance between the humors, and treatment was aimed at restoring the balance and reinstating internal harmony.

From Rome to the Renaissance

Scientific investigations continued to flourish in Greece, but in time Rome also became a center of learning. It was in Rome that another great physician, Galen, made his home. During the latter half of the second century A.D., Galen assiduously studied the anatomy of the respiratory system and of the heart, arteries and veins, and wrote some four hundred treatises on medicine. Many of his observations were correct, although a number of his treatises contained some fundamental errors.

The decline of ancient medicine in Europe coincided with the decline of Rome in the fifth century A.D.. These were the Dark Ages, beleaguered with epidemics and plagues, which doctors were powerless to cure. There was thus a move against the Greek approach to medicine based on reason and empirical experiments, and a resurgence of superstitious practices.

Although the Middle Ages saw the foundation of the universities, and of guilds, pharmacies and hospitals, for several hundred years the growth of rational medicine progressed very slowly. The widespread despair caused by the interminable succession of epidemics was fertile ground for all types of quackery. It was not until the Renaiss-

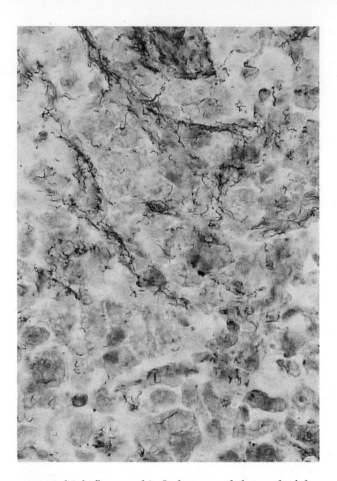

veloped. Early microscopists could then see for the first time the tiny blood capillaries (confirming Harvey's discovery), the intricate structure of the organs of the body, and the microscopic organisms. Physiological experiments began to unravel the functions of the heart, liver and lungs.

Eighteenth-century Endeavors

The eighteenth century saw the emergence of physicians in something like the modern style. Their practice was based more firmly on biological knowledge and, under the influences of Thomas Sydenham (sometimes referred to as the English Hippocrates), the importance of observation at the bedside, and the patient-doctor relationship, was reaffirmed.

At the same time there were the first signs of progress in the field of mental health care. Up until then, mental illness or insanity was linked with demonic possession or witchcraft, and sufferers were apallingly treated; many were strapped up and locked away under brutish conditions. Some also came to be used as harmless objects of fun and were exhibited at fairs.

At this time the Italian Giovanni Morgagni (1682–1771) founded the science of modern pathology. He studied the anatomical difference between the healthy and unhealthy body and showed that anatomical alterations were the source of the functional alterations felt by patients as symptoms. He asserted that a crucial way of improving the practice of medicine was for doctors to compare the findings of autopsies, which revealed the true nature of illness, with the diagnosis they made from bedside observation during the life of the patient. Nevertheless, although this was an era of many brilliant clinicians, and scientists, it was also the heyday of charlatans.

The eighteenth century is commonly regarded as the golden age of quackery. One of the most infamous in duping the authorities was a woman named Joanna Stephens. She sold her prescription for the treatment of gallstones to the British Parliament for five thousand pounds. It was made of crushed snails, powdered eggshells, burned berries, soap and honey.

Another striking example of quackery was the ''Celestial Bed'' — an invention of the Scotsman

ance, which flowered in Italy toward the end of the fifteenth century, that the more rational and less mystical Greek attitude was restored.

The man who is celebrated as the father of anatomy was a Flemish physician named Andreas Vesalius. His monumental work *De humani corporis fabrica*, published in 1543, presented a complete study of the structure of the human body. Vesalius pointed out the many fundamental errors of Galen, whose anatomical studies were performed almost wholly on animals and extrapolated to humans. Vesalius forcefully asserted the need to conduct human dissections.

In some respects, the Renaissance *was* an age of enlightenment. But even while the studies of anatomy and physiology were advancing rapidly during the seventeenth century, medical practice still clung to many old Hippocratic and Galenic ideas. Finally, the Englishman William Harvey (1578–1657) discovered the circulation by showing that arterial blood flowed from the left side of the heart to all parts of the body, returning to the right side in the great veins. From there the venous blood was pumped to the lungs and back to the left side of the heart as arterial or oxygenated blood.

During the 1600s microscopes were also de-

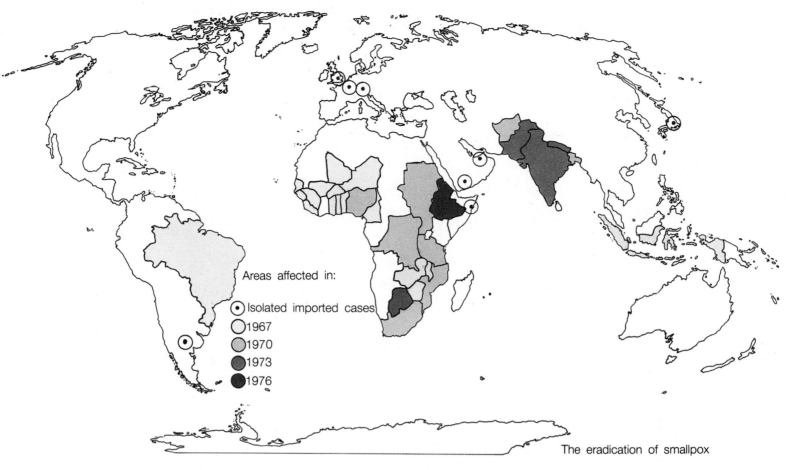

Areas affected in:

⊙ Isolated imported cases
◯ 1967
◯ 1970
◯ 1973
● 1976

The eradication of smallpox

James Graham. The bed, twelve feet long and nine feet wide, was supported by forty pillars of brilliant glass in a "Temple of Health," based on the Aesculapian design. The dome of the bed was infused with balms and spices, and further "therapeutic force" was provided by magnets.

The idea that magnetism could be exploited in the treatment of disease was not new, but the greatest figure in the history of medicine to have based his therapies on the purported healing powers of "animal magnetism" was surely Franz Anton Mesmer (1734–1815). His patients, having waited weeks for an appointment, were arranged around a bath of dilute sulphuric acid from which curved iron bars protruded. In dim lights and perfumed air, patients grasped the bars and formed a circle waiting for the scarlet-robed Mesmer to touch each person; surprisingly often he was able to induce a hypnotic state — hence the derivation of the word mesmerism.

Another eighteenth-century revival was the theory that "like cures like," advanced by the German practitioner Samuel Hahnemann (1755–1843) and termed homeopathic theory. Homeopathy still has its adherents. In fact, Hahnemann's homeopathic followers founded a medical school in his name that exists to this day in Philadelphia. Hahnemann had noted that a dose of quinine produced a fever that was similar to the fever of malaria — the disease that quinine was used to treat. From this he postulated that very great dilutions of drugs would cure symptoms that the same drug, at high doses, would produce. As one famous British pharmacologist remarked, however, the recommended dilutions were so great that the tinctures or herbal remedies would contain only a few molecules of active drug in a sphere the size of the earth. By coincidence Hahnemann's introductory manifesto of homeopathy was published in the same year that Edward Jenner implanted cowpox into a boy to see if it gave him an immunity to smallpox.

Jenner (1749–1823) was a country doctor in Gloucester, England, where it was common knowledge that milkmaids infected with cowpox were immune to smallpox — a disease which claimed an estimated sixty million lives in eighteenth century Europe. After twenty years of systematic work, Jenner carried out his decisive experiment on May 14, 1796. He extracted the contents of a pustule on the hand of a milkmaid infected with cowpox, and injected it into the arm of a healthy

13

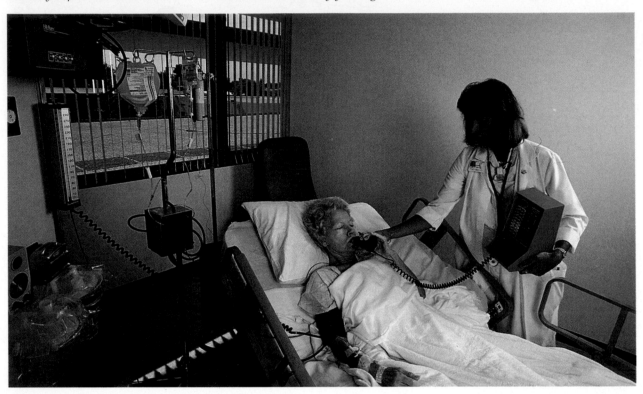

eight-year-old boy. The child suffered no ill effects from the cowpox inoculation, and six weeks later Jenner inoculated him with material from human smallpox pustules; the boy did not catch smallpox. Vaccination, as the technique came to be called, heralded the beginning of the field of preventive medicine, but it was to be a long time before the superstitions and criticisms of this effective and safe practice were to be finally dispelled, and another hundred years before the mechanisms of immunity were finally understood.

The Pain Killers

Medical knowledge grew throughout the nineteenth century, particularly in the fields of physiology and pathology, and the art of medical care gained some benefits from the new discoveries. At this time, however, the horizons of surgery were limited because the problems of pain, sepsis, hemorrhage and post-surgical shock had yet to be solved. Of these, pain was the greatest handicap to the surgeon's task.

The prolonged failure of physicians to find ways to remove or reduce pain presents one of the most baffling stories in medical history. That certain plants could be prescribed as painkillers had been known since the earliest days of medicine. Opium was used as early as in the third millennium B.C.; and the effects of Indian hemp (cannabis) were known in ancient times in the east and used by surgeons in China in the second century A.D.

Sleep-inducing drugs were in use throughout the Middle Ages and into the Renaissance. The great physician Paracelsus popularized laudanum, a tincture of opium. Even William Shakespeare made reference to the use of narcotics: "Not poppy, not mandragora, not all the drowsy spirits of the world shall ever medicine thee to that sweet sleep." Yet in eighteenth-century Europe, a patient would be thought lucky to receive anything to kill the agonizing pain of a surgical operation — and at best would be given a large dose of alcohol.

Nitrous oxide gas was disovered in 1772 by the British chemist Joseph Priestley; in 1800 his compatriot Humphrey Davy described its analgesic and exhilarating effects. Davy had tried the drug on himself, and later on his friends (including the poets Samuel Coleridge and William Wordsworth), but his suggestion that it might be advantageous for use in surgical operations was ignored. Davy's pupil Michael Faraday, who also described the painkilling effects of the gas, was to discover the anesthetic properties of ether in 1818. It was not until the mid-nineteenth century that modern surgical anesthesia began to be practiced — and bitter controversy then arose over who actually discovered its use.

During the 1840s it became fashionable for young men to get together to inhale nitrous oxide or "laughing gas" for convivial purposes. The American Crawford Long (1815–1873) noticed that ether had the same effects as nitrous oxide, and he introduced it as an alternative "tipple" to his friends in Georgia. Long observed that both he and his friends would sustain falls and blows while under the influence of ether, with no later recollection of pain being felt at the time of such accidents. In 1842 Long painlessly removed a tumor from a friend's neck while ether was administered through a towel. The friend felt no pain.

Possibly from fear of censure, Long did not publish his results. At the same time, however, Horace Wells — a dentist from Hartford, Connecticut — began to use nitrous oxide for dental operations. Later he gave a demonstration of his tested technique in the Massachusetts General Hospital, but unfortunately for some reason his equipment failed and the patient yelled in agony. A former assistant of Wells, William Morton, persisted with the idea and when at Harvard Medical School carried out further experiments with ether to test its anesthetic properties. In 1846 Morton successfully demonstrated a painless tooth extraction and a tumor removal with patients under the influence of ether, and from that moment the reputation and use of anesthetics spread rapidly.

Chloroform, another anesthetic, introduced shortly after ether, was first used medically in 1847 by a Scottish obstetrician, John Simpson. He used it, as he had ether, to relieve the pain of childbirth. A few years later this anesthetic received royal assent — Queen Victoria delivered her seventh son, Prince Leopold, under chloroform anesthesia. However, more recently it has been discovered

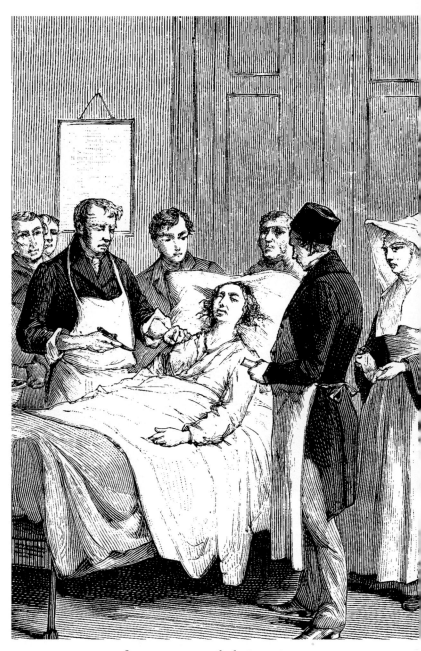

Surgery was once the last resort, a "kill or cure" treatment for conditions that would otherwise be fatal. Pain, shock, loss of blood and infection were the surgeon's greatest enemies. Experiments in the early nineteenth century showed that, for some patients undergoing minor surgery, pain could be relieved by hypnosis. With the development of anesthesia and the realization of the importance of hygiene, clinical mortality rates declined rapidly.

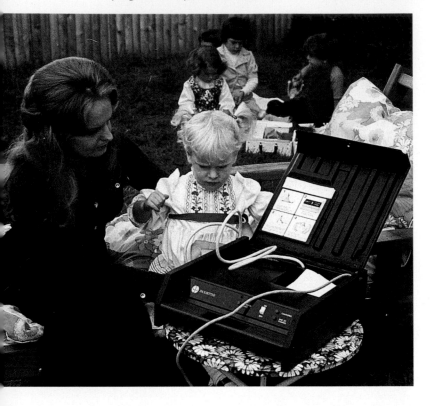

that chloroform has side effects on the liver and heart, and ether irritates the respiratory tract; nitrous oxide is less toxic, but does not produce sufficiently deep sleep or the muscle relaxation necessary for longer operations.

In time, new anesthetics were developed. Barbiturates came into general use in the early years of the twentieth century, and are still used today for the induction of anesthesia. Local anesthetics, such as cocaine, were first described in 1884, whereas drugs such as curare and succinylcholine, which produce muscle relaxation necessary for some major operations, were not introduced into anesthetics until after 1945. In 1929 cyclopropane was introduced, but this had the disadvantage (like ether) of being explosively inflammable and not safe for use in modern operating theaters.

As anesthetists have often pointed out, it is chiefly because of their success in the development of new anesthetics and of new techniques in using them that surgery has been able to make its most spectacular advances. Some feel, indeed, that surgeons tend to take too much credit for achievements that should be shared.

Next to Godliness

The story of delays in introducing a germ-free environment (asepsis) to Western medicine is similar to that concerning anesthesia. Physicians in the ancient civilizations of Babylon and Egypt had been obsessed by cleanliness, and even up until the Renaissance physicians had recognized the need for cleanliness in aiding the natural healing of wounds. But this important idea gradually disappeared from the doctors' set of guidelines. When the poor were crowded into hospitals, bringing their dirt with them, demands for cleanliness in the operating room may have seemed somewhat pedantic.

Maternity wards provided the starting point for the development of modern aseptic techniques. A Hungarian obstetrician, Ignaz Semmelweiss (1818–1865), was appalled at the number of women who died from puerperal fever, a persistent fever that affected them soon after childbirth. He noted that there were fewer deaths in a maternity ward attended by midwives than in a ward attended by the obstetrician. He put this together with another fact he had noted; each morning, before commencing their ward work, obstetricians performed autopsies on the patients who had recently died. Midwives never attended autopsies. Eventually Semmelweiss realized that puerperal fever was simply a manifestation of septicemia (blood poisoning), and became convinced that the infection was transmitted by the doctors from the corpses to the women in labor. He issued strict orders that hands must be thoroughly washed after each medical examination and that the wards must be cleaned with calcium chloride (a disinfectant). Within two years, the mortality rate in the maternity ward attributable to puerperal fever dropped almost to zero.

Semmelweiss reported to the Medical Society in Vienna that puerperal fever was a septicemia, but his communication was opposed by his colleagues and he was dismissed from his post. He returned to Hungary, were he continued to improve his aseptic techniques and where he succeeded in eradicating puerperal sepsis from the old hospital

The computer is a new and powerful device for probing the mechanisms of the human body. This colorful image is of a protein molecule, created by computer graphics from an analysis of its complex chemical composition, also carried out by a computer. The molecule — in this case the major component of a muscle fiber — can be turned through three dimensions on screen, giving researchers a complete picture of its structure.

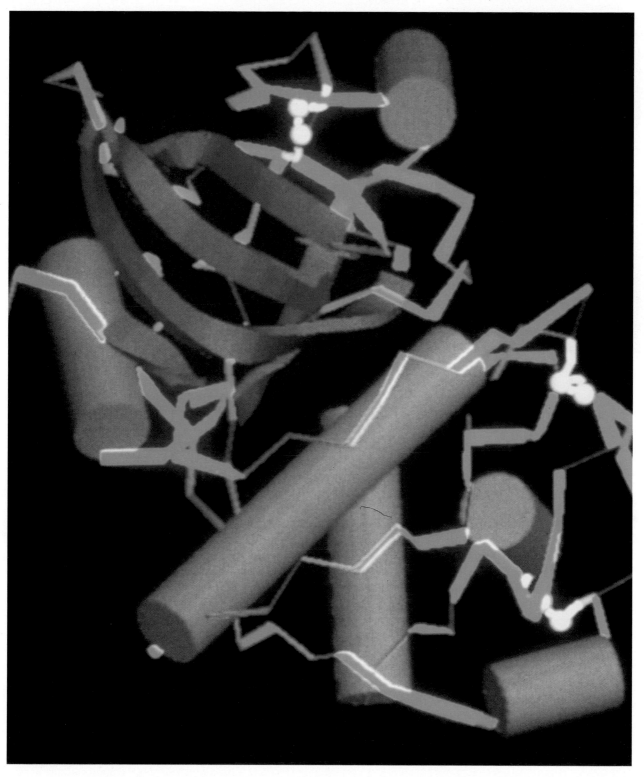

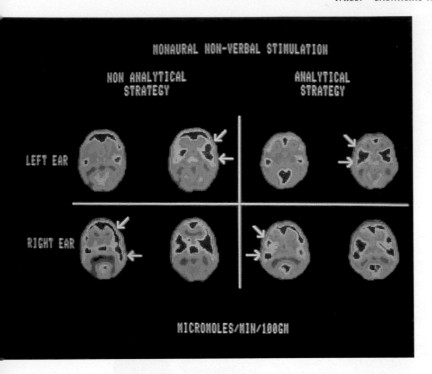

of St. Rock. Meanwhile in Vienna, in his absence, students and doctors once more stopped washing and disinfecting their hands — and the death rate among newly-delivered women soared back to its previous level. Semmelweiss eventually published his ideas in 1861; his book stands as one of the epoch-making works of medical literature.

At the time when the work of Semmelweiss was rejected by the Viennese medical establishment, the English surgeon Joseph Lister (1827–1912), who was already familiar with Pasteur's work on microorganisms, began to develop the practice of antisepsis. Determined to reduce postoperative infections and gangrene, he adopted one of three measures shown by Pasteur to inhibit the growth of microorganisms, namely disinfection. In 1865 Lister used a variety of disinfectants before settling on carbolic acid (phenol) which, in conjunction with meticulous cleanliness, produced striking results. Most of Lister's patients survived surgery and recovered within a short period of time. The antiseptic method caught on at once, and spread throughout the medical world. Lister received many of the highest honors, including a knighthood from Queen Victoria and a peerage.

The practice of antisepsis was followed by asepsis, in which the surgeon's aim was to exclude microorganisms totally from the operating room, instead of destroying them with disinfectants. Asepsis made use of another of Pasteur's combative measures — heat. In 1886 the German Ernst von Bergmann introduced sterilization of dressing using superheated steam under pressure in an autoclave, which quickly became standard equipment for the operating theater. Four years later the American W. S. Halstead initiated the use of sterile rubber gloves during operations.

A Great Battle on a Small Scale

At about this time, another significant advance occurred in the history of medicine. The microscope was brought to an advanced stage of development. This allowed the study of the structure and function of the body at the cellular level, and pathological studies proliferated. The greatest name in this field in the nineteenth century was that of the German pathologist Rudolph Virchow (1821–1902) who, through autopsies, the collection of pathological specimens and pioneering microscopy, opened the way for the foundation of microbiology. From his work Virchow showed that the macroscopic and microscopic changes occurring in diseased organisms were no more than the reaction of cells to the causative agents of the disease. The disease could be identified by looking at the appropriate cells of the patient. Although Virchow did not identify the agents responsible for many diseased states, he did dispel the ancient concept that disease is caused by imbalance of the humors, which had been passed down through medicine since ancient times.

It was Louis Pasteur, born in France in 1822, who first showed that disease could be caused, and spread, by microorganisms. His important studies did not begin until he became director of scientific studies in the Paris Ecole Normale in 1857, where he started to study the process of fermentation. Pasteur found that fermentation was caused by living microorganisms (not merely the chemical breakdown of yeasts). He also discovered that the decomposition of wine to vinegar, and of milk to lactic acid, were caused by reactions brought about by living microorganisms.

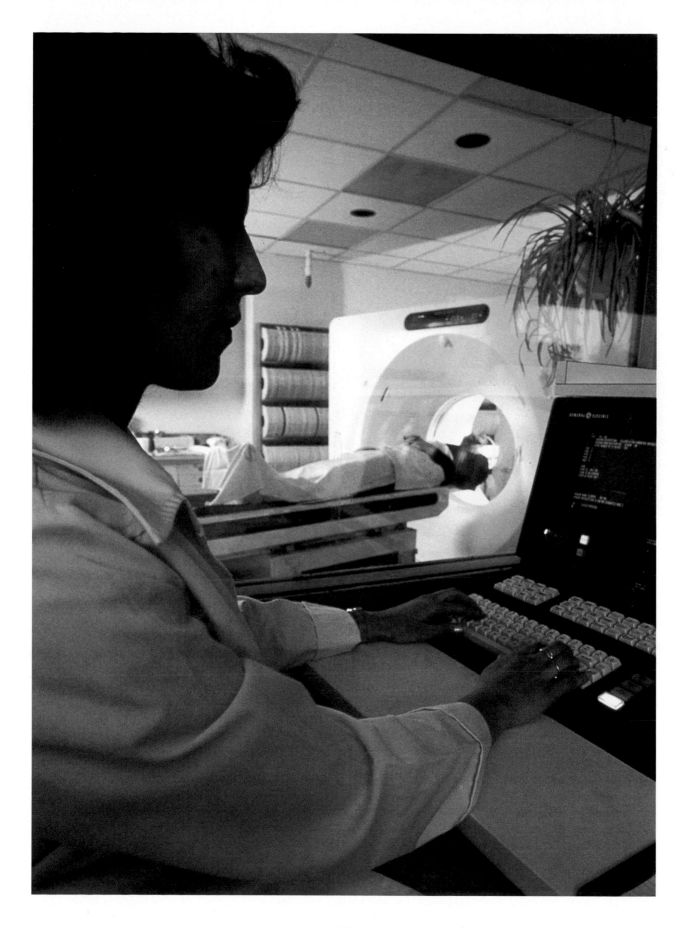

A laser beam cuts tissue at a precisely-defined area of the brain — a specimen is used here for demonstration purposes. Lasers have three principal advantages over conventional surgical tools. Firstly,

the beam of high-intensity light can be directed to an accuracy of under one-thousandth of an inch; secondly, laser light is completely sterile; and thirdly, the laser seals the tiny capillaries around the affected area,

preventing blood loss. For many routine eye operations, such as the removal of cataracts, and for certain types of neurological surgery, the laser has replaced the scalpel in modern medicine.

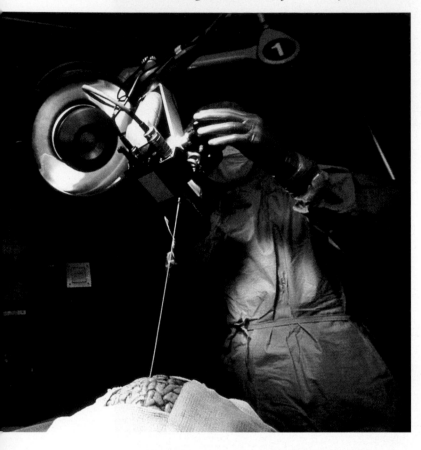

was the first drug shown to have a benefit in treating syphilis. Ehrlich also provided the groundwork for immunology by showing that serum taken from the blood of an animal infected with a microorganism had a specific antitoxic effect on the same disease-producing substances.

It is now known that the effects of such a serum results from the action of specific antibodies manufactured by the body in neutralizing the antigens of the invading microorganisms. It therefore followed that there were two possible means of protecting an individual against the effects of pathogenic organisms. One was active immunization, in which microorganisms of reduced virulence were injected into the bloodstream and the individual manufactured antibodies in response to the injected microorganisms. The other was passive immunization, in which antibodies in the serum from an animal that had previously been infected conferred immunity on the person into whom the serum was injected.

Two further victories in the war against infection were the recognition of the role taken by insects in the transmission of disease (for example the mosquito in malaria), and the identification and study of viruses.

Early chemical agents against disease, such as Ehrlich's Salvarsan, were toxic and not highly effective. But in 1935 the first sulfonamide drugs were introduced. Since then these antibacterial compounds have constituted an important part of the modern pharmacopoeia. The greatest landmark in the development of antibacterial drugs was the discovery of penicillin by the team led by the British bacteriologist Alexander Fleming. His historic chance observation was made in 1928, when he noticed that contamination of a culture of staphylococci bacteria with the fungus *Penicillium notatum* caused the bacterial colonies around the fungus to disappear.

In Oxford, Howard Florey and Ernst Chain pursued investigations, and succeeded in developing a way to acquire sufficient quantities of penicillin to begin animal experiments with it in 1940. Within a few years, it was being produced on a large scale in the United States; huge vats, containing thousands of gallons of nutrient solution were used for culturing the penicillin-producing fungus.

Invited by wine producers to investigate the souring of wine, Pasteur discovered that heating the wine to about 140°F for a short time did not affect the quality of the wine but killed the bacteria responsible for the formation of vinegar. Thereafter, similar heating was applied to other consumer products, such as milk, in a process that came to be known as pasteurization in honor of its inventor. Pasteur later applied this technique therapeutically: he isolated the bacteria that cause anthrax and rabies and, after their partial destruction by heat, he used these less virulent preparations as vaccines to produce immunization.

The founder of chemotherapy and of immunology was Paul Ehrlich (1845–1915), who discovered that dyes and other chemicals selectively attach themselves to specific microorganisms and so destroy them. The drug Salvarsan, which was much more toxic to bacteria than to the cells of the human body, was one of his discoveries in 1910. It

Asklepios to Paracelsus
Early Frontiersmen

Throughout history there have been many eminent medical men whose work has entirely changed the course of medical knowledge and practice. Few, however, could claim to have had an influence that lasted for centuries. But, from the time of the ancient Greeks, Asklepios (if he ever existed) and Hippocrates certainly did, as during the Roman age did Galen, and as much later the pre-Renaissance physician Paracelsus also did.

Asklepios — known to the Romans as Aesculapius — is mentioned by Homer as a medical expert present at the siege of Troy. By the classical age of the ancient Greeks, however, he was accorded the worship due to a deity in shrines attended by robed priests.

Hippocrates is said to have studied at the Temple of Asklepios at Cos in the mid-fifth century B.C., and was a contemporary of Plato who described his medical ability with some awe. So venerated did he become during his lifetime that within a century after his death all the medical knowledge and philosophy then available was assembled in a single work titled the *Collection* to which Hippocrates' name was attached. The *Collection* included the famous Hippocratic Oath, many ethical

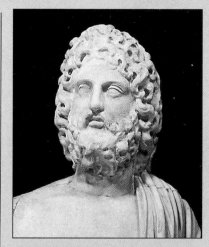

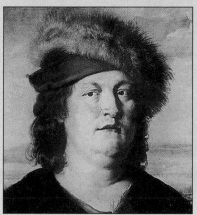

points of which remain morally (if not legally) in force today.

Nearly five centuries after the completion of the *Collection*, the well-traveled physician Galen settled in Rome and began giving medical lectures and demonstrating his new techniques of treatment, incidentally becoming also the confidant of no fewer than three successive Roman Emperors

(including Marcus Aurelius). His skill lay mainly in anatomical and physiological study; his public dissections were revolutionary in that he sought to explain how the body works as much as to treat wounds and diseases. If Hippocrates can be said to have founded the art of healing, Galen can reasonably be said to have founded the science of examination.

Why Paracelsus should have become so famous in the early 1500s — and why his name remains celebrated even now — is something of a mystery. Superstitious, ignorant of some of the medical advances of his own time, and inaccurate in observation, he nevertheless wrote many much-used works on treatments, involving especially mineral baths, tinctures and extracts, and was both lauded and derided by his contemporaries. One aspect of his character may be evident in the fact that he chose to be known as Paracelsus (although his true name was Theophrastus Bombastus von Hohenheim). In his emphasis on the efficacy of minerals to health, however, he was in some respects a forerunner of those who today strongly advocate the benefits of trace elements in diet and metabolic functions.

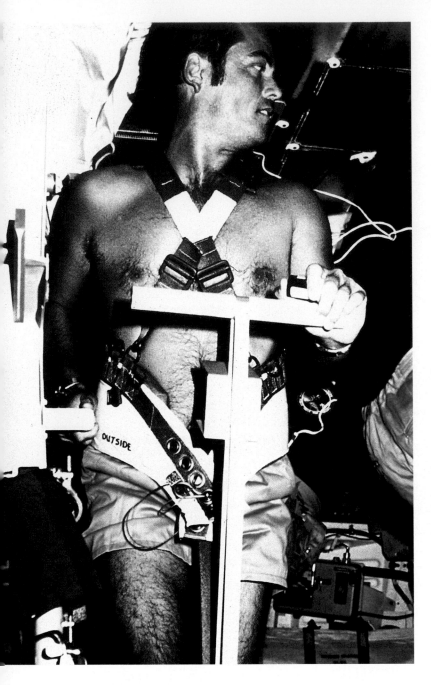

The conquest of space was arguably the ultimate technological achievement of our century. Critics of the space program argue that there are problems of disease and poverty on earth that warrant more attention and money, but space research has also brought benefits in social and medical fields. For example, studies of astronauts submitted to long-term weightlessness have provided new insight into the way calcium is metabolized in the body.

The emergence of drug-resistant bacterial strains was first noted with sulfonamide treatment and then with penicillin. For this reason, other antibiotics such as streptomycin (1944), chloramphenicol (1947) and aureomycin (1948) were developed, as were methods for the synthesis of new variants of penicillin.

Today effective antibiotic drugs are available for the treatment of nearly all bacterial diseases. Viruses, on the other hand, are unaffected by antibiotics; the best defense against them is a good level of antibodies, normally produced by active immunization, although antiviral drugs continue to be developed. From Paul Ehrlich's early work, immunology and chemotherapy have gone far beyond their original uses in the fight against infectious diseases. Chemotherapy for treating cancer and making transplant surgery possible are but two examples of the continuing importance of immunology in medicine.

Mens Sana . . .

The branch of medicine that took the most time to arouse itself from the torpor of centuries was psychiatry, the treatment of people who are mentally ill. The nineteenth century had been a melancholy period indeed for mental patients, and the ideas of William Tuke and Philippe Pinel had been disregarded. One name that stands out in this period is that of Dorothea Dix. Appalled by the conditions of mental institutions in Massachusetts, she managed to rouse public concern for mental patients and the fact that they were locked away with inmates of workhouses and prisons. Unfortunately, however, this led to an even worse fate for those classified as insane, because they were then locked away in special asylums with even smaller likelihood of release.

The vivid descriptions of life in asylums, portrayed in Clifford Beer's biography *A Mind That Found Itself* (1908), ultimately led to the foundation of the National Committee for Mental Hygiene in the United States. This went some way to improving mental hospitals, but the improvement was short-lived — because the criterion by which mental illness was considered tolerable in public was changed. The unfortunate result was that even more patients were institutionalized.

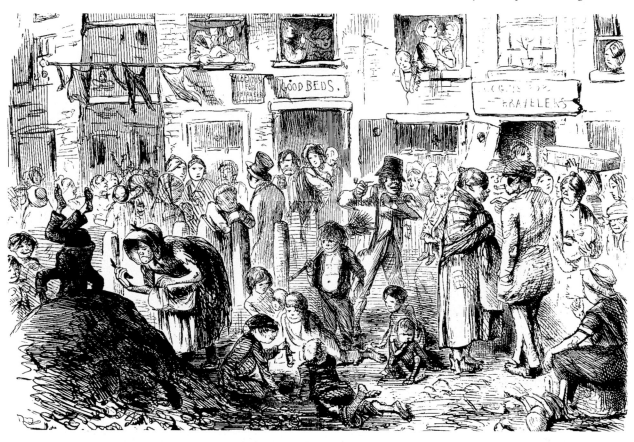

In the late nineteenth century and the early twentieth centuries two forms of treatment for the mentally sick were available — psychotherapy and drugs. Stemming from mesmerism, hypnosis was adopted as a means of helping patients to release repressed emotions and recollections; this "catharsis" was found to help the neuroses of the mentally ill. Sigmund Freud in Vienna began his investigations into psychoanalysis and the unconscious mind by using hypnosis, but he later abandoned this technique when he found that a hypnotic state was not necessary for seeking the repressed experiences and problems of the patient. The Swiss psychiatrist Carl Jung and the Austrian Alfred Adler were disciples of Freud, but headed their own groups. Nevertheless, the divisions between them were, in principle, not great. All were analysts who sought to persuade patients to talk about their neuroses and thereby acquire insights that would enable them to cope with them.

Psychotherapy, like behavioral therapy, was time-consuming and costly, and was certainly no treatment for agitated psychotic or schizophrenic patients. For them the only form of treatment up until the mid-twentieth century was sedation by such drugs as laudanum (tincture of opium) and barbiturates, which were first developed as anesthetics in the early twentieth century. Electroconvulsive therapy (ECT), commonly known as shock therapy, followed.

The real revolution in the treatment of the mentally ill came in the 1950s when the tranquilizer chlorpromazine (Largactil) was introduced. This drug had the effect of inducing a tranquil state without sedation, and was therefore effective in controlling psychotic symptoms without, literally, putting the patient to sleep. One major outcome of this discovery and of the development of other similar drugs was a dramatic change in the care of the mentally ill. Mental hospitals began to adopt

Disease-producing microorganisms, which enter the body via the skin, digestive or respiratory tracts, or via the sexual organs, have historically been the major causes of ill health. They remain so in the poorer

countries of the world. Self-inflicted diseases — such as those caused by smoking, overindulgence in alcohol, poor diet and lack of exercise — are now the causes of premature death in the developed nations of North

America, Europe and Australasia. Accidents and traumas also continue to take their toll, whereas the incidence of congenital disease decreases in populations when wealth and living standards rise.

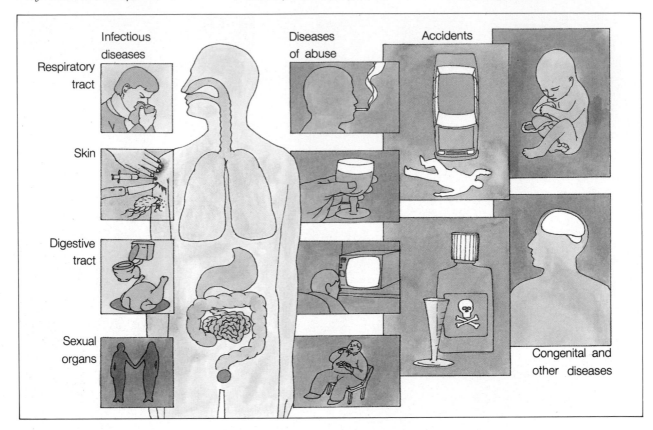

an "Open Door" system; a regime of community care rather than institutionalized care became a reality for many patients. However, tranquilizers and similar drugs do not cure mental illness; they simply mask the symptoms. Until more is understood about the organic cause of psychiatric disturbances, researchers have few clues to guide them in developing chemotherapies that might counteract any chemical imbalance and restore the "normal" function of the brain.

The working of the brain as a whole organ remains largely a mystery. It is known to be an incredibly complex network with billions of nerve cells and trillions of connections. It is also known that the messages pass through the network as electrical impulses, but that chemical activities are needed to pass the impulse from cell to cell. Certain parts of the brain form different controlling centers for different functions, but interconnections are manifold. What is not known is how these different parts interconnect. Just how do we

control memory, emotions and behavior, and how does the brain integrate these functions in order to direct appropriate responses to the environment? Because the brain is so complex an organ, it is not difficult to appreciate how a dysfunction in just one controlling center could be the cause of inappropriate responses, abnormal behavior and mental illness.

Any defect in the integrative role of the brain can also be the cause of psychosomatic illness, in which a change of mental state induces a physical change in bodily functions. Although belief in psychosomatic medicine has waxed and waned through the centuries, the importance of a patient's emotional condition in the etiology of disease states has recently gained some acceptance. Chronic forms of stress seem to be particularly relevant in this respect. Medical practitioners are beginning to recognize the need for treatments that are not simply directed at a physical cure. Forms of relaxation and meditation, for example, are becoming acknowledged as potentially valuable elements of health care.

. . . in Corpore Sano

The word "medicine" is most commonly associated with hospital wards and doctors' clinics, to which sick people go for treatment. The importance of preventive medicine in maintaining health is often forgotten. One major aspect of preventive medicine, already mentioned, is immunization against disease. There are, however, more subtle and perhaps more cost-effective forms of preventive medicine that are related to public hygiene, poverty, general health care and health education.

From the earliest times, societies have recognized a need to protect the health of their citizens. One of the fundamental principles of ancient Hebrew medicine, for instance, was hygiene, based on Jewish doctrines. Hand washing before and after meals, hygienic "purity" for women during and just after menstruation, and cleansing of the sick were all part of religious duties, and every synagogue was built with a ritual bath. The Romans were also concerned with public hygiene. They built sewers and drainage systems for waste disposal, and great aqueducts to carry fresh water to the city of Rome. They also drained marshy areas close to urban settlements in order to eliminate mosquitoes. But the later lapse in interest in the early achievements in this field meant that there was little or no defense against such lethal epidemics as the Black Death, and in the Middle Ages and afterward the flourishing growth of crowded walled cities caused a further lowering in the standards of personal and communal hygiene, and led consequently to widespread disease.

One of the greatest problems of these cities was the disposal of excreta. An answer was provided by the Englishman John Harrington (1561–1612), who invented the water closet which enabled excreta to be flushed away into cesspools. Although the contents of these cesspools tended to soak into the surrounding soil and pollute wells and rivers, in 1695 his device was carefully described in his report entitled *New discourse of a stale subject, called the Metamorphosis of Ajax*. ("Ajax" was a pun on "a jakes," the old word for "privy.") This prepared the way for general public health.

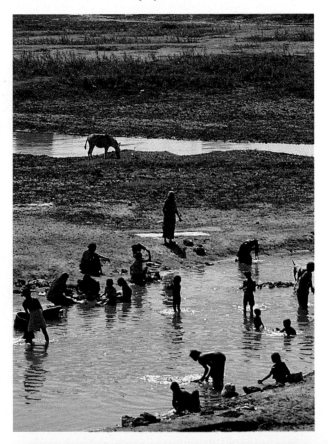

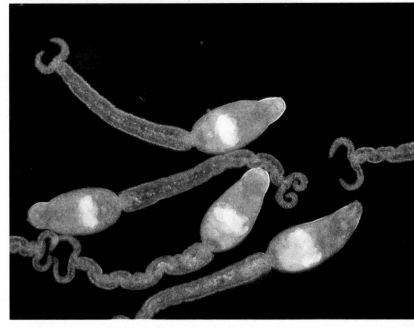

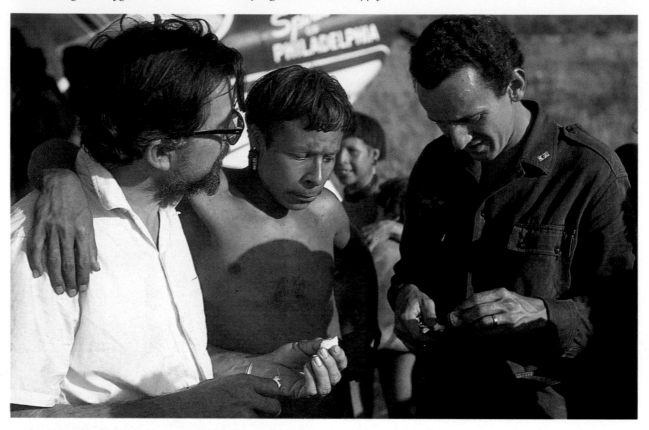

The Industrial Revolution produced hundreds of thousands of badly built hovels, in which ill health and disease were favored because of the overcrowding and the lack of ventilation and light. In England in 1803 the repeal of the window tax (by which the government levied a charge for each window in a building) helped slightly with light and ventilation, but in the smoky industrial towns there was already little enough natural light, and in addition poor nutrition was symptomatic of the poverty in urban areas.

Modern Health Organizations

The most energetic advocate of public health laws was Edwin Chadwick, secretary of the Poor Law Commission in England and a persistent campaigner for the eradication of poverty as a way to prevent sickness. His plans involved a considerable expenditure of public money, and it is therefore not surprising that he accumulated many influential enemies. In fact, in the 1850s he was given a liberal pension on condition that, as he ruefully commented, he would "leave dirt and disease alone."

Years after Chadwick's death, almost all the measures he had recommended had to be introduced piecemeal by later governments. Thus during the latter part of the nineteenth century, great strides were made in improving the physical environment and reducing poverty. Even so, many of the great public health concepts advanced in the nineteeth and early twentieth centuries failed to be implemented. It was not until well into the present century that general health care and preventive medicine were provided by established health services in Europe and North America.

In his history of medicine in the United States, written in the early 1930s, the Swiss medical historian Henry Sigerist remarked on the contrast between what is known about disease and what is actually done about it. His analysis of the first part of this century emphasizes the contrast between the remarkable advances in curative medicine and the failure to put them into practice. So even as medicine pointed with pride to the number of communicable diseases that were being brought under its control, thousands of people were still dying from them each year — and still are dying from them today in the developing countries.

At the present time, in almost all of the world's developed countries, there exist insurance schemes, free or subsidized health services responsible for maintaining state health regulations. Among the earliest regulations to be introduced were those concerning children, and today it is one of the basic principles of most societies that children should not work and should be provided with free education as well as complete medical protection. Vaccination programs have resulted in the eradication of many diseases, and careful observations of children through their early years can help to monitor health and protect against abnormalities in development.

On a worldwide scale the provision of health services is the responsibility of the World Health Organization (WHO), which provides extensive health education and medical aid. Despite this, one of the greatest problems facing medicine today is that, in the underdeveloped countries, hundreds of thousands of people still die of malnutrition, starvation or diseases for which there has long been a cure.

In the modern world physicians find themselves facing many new problems that are the direct product of a rapidly evolving way of life. The effects of the strains and stresses of modern urban society on health and disease represent a still largely unknown factor, and psychiatric diseases present medicine with some of its most perplexing problems. At the same time modern drugs, surgery and special nursing can successfully prolong a healthy and normal life, and so care of the aged becomes more important. And while medicine can prolong the life of many patients with serious disabilities, so the welfare and occupation of these patients is another task for both medicine and society as a whole. Against this backcloth it must be remembered that diseases are continually evolving and changing, presenting new challenges even to the technology of modern medicine.

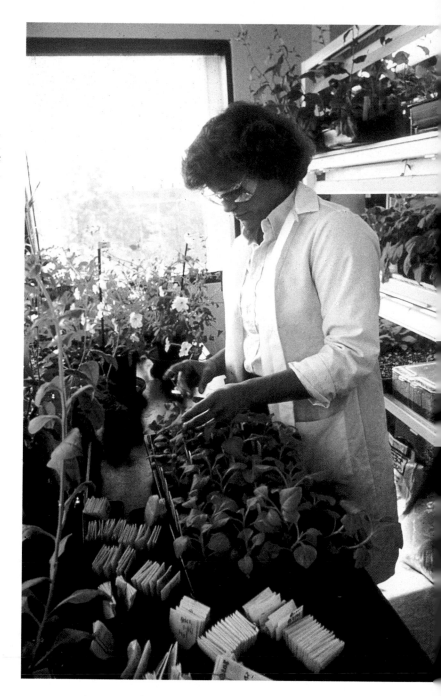

The major drug manufacturing companies are continually developing and testing new products. Plant extracts continue to be one of the most important sources of new drugs. Once the active ingredient is isolated, it may be synthesized by the company's biochemists. However, it is sometimes more economic, as with many alkaloid drugs, for example, to extract the substance from its natural source.

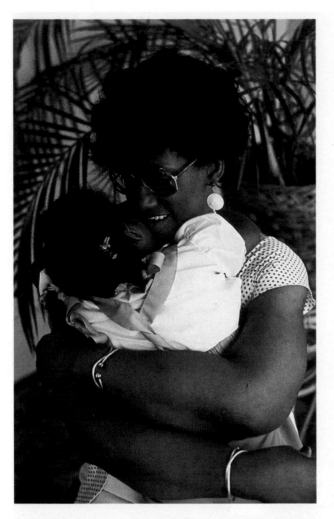

Unfortunately, the AIDS virus has spread through a part of the population notoriously difficult to control. Drug addicts — especially those who use intravenous drugs such as heroin — are very likely to become infected if they use dirty or shared syringes and needles. In many parts of the world heroin addiction and prostitution also go hand in hand. The money from sex is spent on drugs, and the need to make large sums of money leads to prostitution. This vicious circle means that some prostitutes are now AIDS carriers.

AIDS can be contracted through homosexual relations and has been dubbed the "gay plague." But it can also be transmitted by heterosexual contact, and many unsuspecting individuals have now picked up the virus. Studies on American soldiers stationed in Europe have detected the first few people infected in this way.

And there is yet another great difficulty: what can be done about all apparently healthy AIDS carriers? Until penicillin effectively eliminated chronic infection with syphilis, most American states required blood tests for syphilis before a

couple could be married. Some still do. Should AIDS tests now be required, and should infected people be prevented from marrying? During an era in which premarital sex is usual, would such measures be at all effective?

Where will an individual's civil rights end and the community's desire to protect itself take over? Insurance companies may demand AIDS tests before issuing policies. AIDS infection may additionally become grounds for divorce, and should children who carry the AIDS virus go to school? If they do, should they be banned from playing sports where they may cut themselves?

The spread of AIDS virus, hepatitis B virus, genital herpes and the rising incidence of cancer of the cervix in young women, all illustrate how changes in social behavior and social organization can change the patterns of disease. The first three of these conditions can be transmitted by sexual intercourse and the fourth is correlated with it. As social mores changed after World War II — partly because penicillin had tamed syphilis and gonorrhea, and effective contraception diminished greatly the risk of pregnancy — a greater number of people had more sexual contacts and different kinds of sexual experiences. The result has been an explosion of sexually-transmitted viruses.

Before the "sexual revolution" most people had only one or a small number of partners in their lifetime. Although all the sexually-transmitted viruses (with the exception of AIDS) were around, they did not spread very far because most people never encountered a carrier; most carriers infected only their own partners. Now that a great number of people each have sexual contact with several partners every year, however, the viruses spread in a way mathematically equivalent to the multiplication of an atomic chain reaction. One infected person gives the virus to many others, who pass it on to their many partners in turn. If there ever comes a time when the majority of people have such an infection, even those who have only one or a few partners are likely to become affected; the only way to avoid sexually-transmitted disease may be celibacy.

Sexual freedom is not the only change in life style related to an increase in disease. The Western diet, which has at least in part contributed to the

A micrograph of skin cells (below) reveals the presence of an opportunistic infection suffered by a person with AIDS. The appearance of a new virus is rare, and has found biologists and genetic engineers

unprepared. Until immunization and treatment become feasible, containing AIDS is the only course of action available. People most at risk include heroin addicts who share syringes with other users.

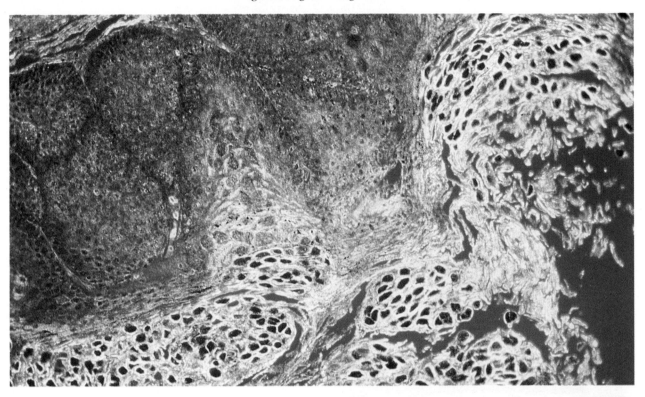

great increase in lifespan this century, has been blamed for the high incidence of heart disease and cancer of the colon. Greater consumption of animal proteins has largely eliminated malnutrition and vitamin deficiency, but has also led to an increase in the consumption of animal fat, which seems to be the culprit here. The recent drastic reduction in many Western countries in lung cancer of men, in heart attacks and in some types of stroke probably results from a decrease in cigarette smoking and an increase in health consciousness, with its emphasis on exercise and a more balanced diet with less animal fat. It is encouraging to see such strong evidence that small changes in behavior can alter the frequency of disease within just one generation.

Vaccination Advances

Genetic engineers have another "trick" that may, in the near future, make many viruses innocuous to humans. Effective immunity to many viruses requires immunization with a "live" virus capable of growing inside normal cells. Part of the protec-

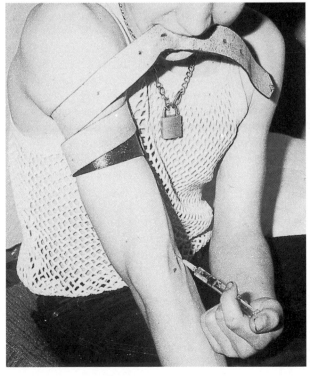

A marriage ceremony can readily be performed at a Las Vegas chapel. The advent of AIDS has led to speculation that marriage might become illegal for anyone found to be carrying the virus.

Progress toward treating AIDS may come from research into drugs already effective in inhibiting herpes infections. These drugs take advantage of an enzyme unique to the herpes virus, shown (right).

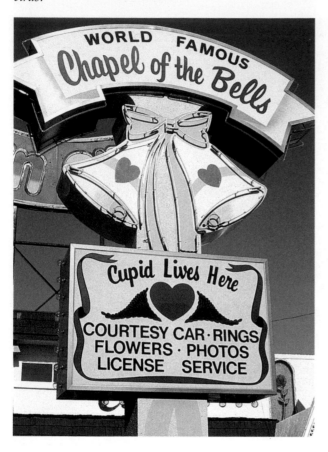

many villages have no electricity and so there is no way to run a freezer. Vaccine must be carried long distances packed in "dry ice" (solid carbon dioxide) and, not surprisingly, in the tropics this does not last very long either. Because there is no electric power there is no way to make more dry ice. This "cold chain" is a major limiting factor in distributing live virus vaccines around the world.

This is where the genetic engineers come in. Scientists in the New York Public Health Department have modified certain viruses to overcome some of these problems. They have cut out part of the genetic material not needed for vaccination and inserted genes from other viruses, including hepatitis B, influenza and rabies. Because the chosen "host" virus is hardy, it can be taken anywhere without a "cold chain." The genetically engineered virus vaccine can immunize against a number of different disease viruses at once.

Both measles and hepatitis B are major diseases that cause health problems worldwide. Measles kills many infants and children in the Third World because it is particularly devastating in the young and malnourished. Hepatitis B virus infects up to half the population of some tropical countries; it produces liver failure and liver cancer. In the West it is largely transmitted by contaminated blood, and is a problem for drug addicts and possibly for medical staff and pathology laboratory workers. An effective vaccine would probably prevent one of the major types of human cancer worldwide.

The Fight Against Cancer

Molecular biology, the science used in genetic engineering, has recently given spectacular insight into how normal cells become cancer cells. In many cases, the abnormality results from a change in one or a few genes that normally control growth and division of cells. These genes were found only in the late 1970s, when scientists learned how to chop up DNA from the few viruses then known to cause cancer. It emerged that the virus had "stolen" a gene from a normal cell and was making it active in the wrong cell, or at the wrong time in the normal complex cycle of events that control cell division. Instead of switching on and off at precisely the right moment for normal developments, the gene remained "on" for too long and the cells

tive effect of immunization depends on the production of specially sensitized white blood cells, called T lymphocytes. Such cells can "recognize" virus proteins only when the viruses are attached to the surface of a living cell. The viral protein forms a complex with one of the proteins on the cell surface called a histocompatibility antigen. The combination is recognized by T lymphocytes as "foreign" and attacked.

Vaccines against viruses can be very difficult to make. In vaccine manufacture, a virus must first be "weakened" in the laboratory so that it cannot cause virulent disease when injected as a vaccine. Then the weak, or attenuated, virus must be purified and packaged. Unfortunately, at room temperature many viruses rapidly lose their ability to infect cells and to stimulate the right sorts of immunity. They must be kept frozen until moments before they are administered. In the United States this seldom poses a problem. But in Africa,

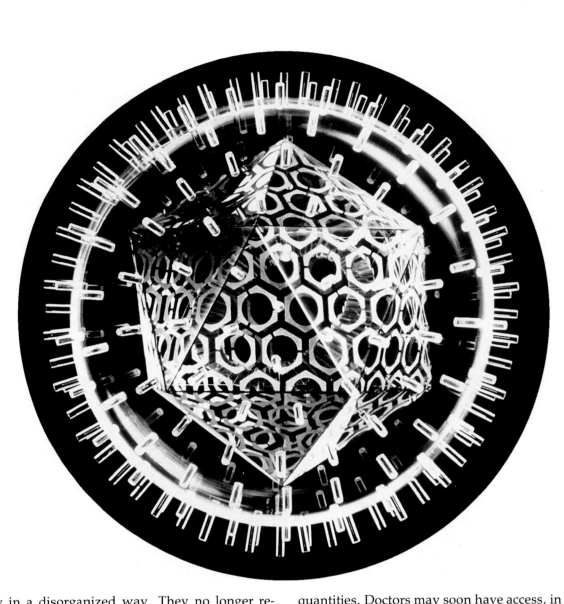

grew in a disorganized way. They no longer responded to the usual "stop" signals that keep normal cells from running wild.

These so-called oncogenes represent a new science — the study of the exact control of cell replication. Scientists foresee a whole new pharmacology of the future involved in studying and producing inhibitors and stimulators of oncogenes and the proteins made by them. Medical science seems to be on the verge of discovering exactly how cancer happens — and of finding out how to reverse or inhibit the process.

New treatments seem to be in store as well. The miracle of molecular biology is that it enables scientists to "read" the structure of any protein molecule made in nature, and copy it by cloning the gene that carries the protein's code.

Suddenly, biologically important molecules — some so rare that scientists have argued about their very existence — could be made in large quantities. Doctors may soon have access, in quantity, to all the critical substances made by the body in response to an infection or tumor.

One such substance is interferon, a protein found in the blood plasma of persons with virus infections. It has the ability of making cells immune to infection. In the last few years the vastly increased availability of interferon has permitted it to be tried against many different types of cancer, offering hope of significant benefit to cancer sufferers. A T-lymphocyte product called interferleukin 2 makes lymphocytes divide and grow. It is being used experimentally to treat cancers and AIDS, and has shown encouraging results. If interferleukin 2 works it will increase the number of lymphocytes in the patient's body, and help to control the disease.

One of the most fascinating of such new molecules is tumor necrosis factor. Before 1984, this was an obscure substance found only in the blood

Prevention is better than cure, and vaccines have improved world health dramatically. The diagram shows those diseases against which inoculation is possible and the main sites of the body each disease attacks.

But new vaccines are urgently needed to combat Third World diseases, to fight cancer, and to stem the AIDS epidemic. Advances in the fields of molecular biology and biotechnology are most likely to provide solutions.

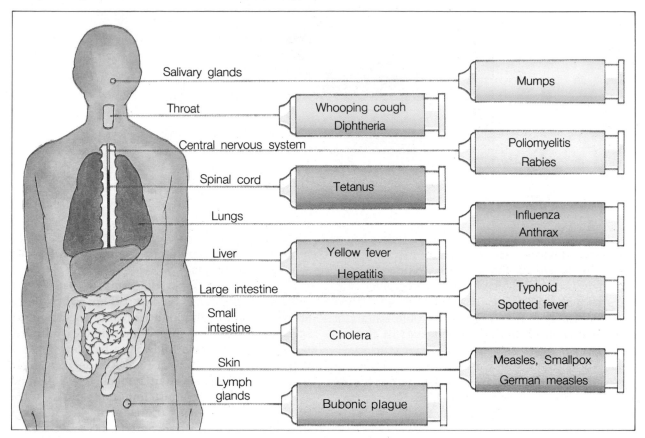

the brain's natural painkillers — chemicals called endorphins and enkephalins — but without the unwanted side effects of current pain relievers. Another possible application is to produce better anticancer agents. Many strategies for cancer treatment rely on drugs that prevent cancer cells from dividing. These compounds bind to DNA and "poison" it so that it cannot be copied. Computer graphics can simulate the shape of DNA with all its twists and turns, and predict which molecules would fit into the structure and make it permanently inactive.

Another approach is to look for molecules that might inhibit specific genes. These drugs would be chosen to bind to active genes and prevent them from being used to make the specific protein that causes a cell to become malignant. A candidate for one such inhibitor is called "antisense RNA," a term applied to an RNA molecule that is the mirror image of a normal RNA molecule. The antisense molecule binds to the normal messenger RNA molecule and prevents it from being translated into protein. The unwanted gene product is thus effectively masked and so cannot function.

Some cancer cells require for growth the presence in the body of natural hormones. Cancer cell growth can be inhibited by surgically removing the hormone-producing gland. But a much better way would be to devise a molecule that mimicked the hormone by binding to the malignant cell and blocking the normal hormone effect. Alternatively, a drug could shut off normal hormone production and "starve" the cancer cell. All of these agents can in principle be designed and "dry tested" on the computer. Only the most promising ones need be sent for trial, saving both time and money. Ultimately, when enough information is in computer banks, it may be possibly to predict which chemical can produce exactly a required side effect long before the drug is physically tested at all.

Modern physical instrumentation has made it possible to take actual pictures of biological mol-

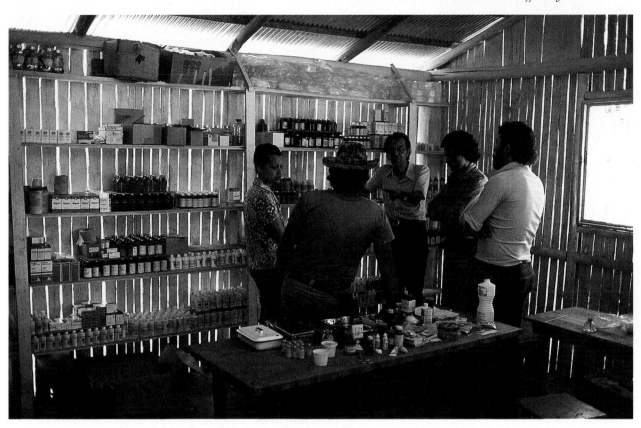

ecules. The first complete high-resolution electron microscope pictures of disease-causing viruses have now appeared. These have revealed that the virus studied (a relative of the many viruses that can cause the common cold) has a large "valley" on one surface. This groove seems to be the place at which the virus attaches to cells before it infects them. Studying the exact composition and shape of the attachment site may make it possible to design a "plug;" a simple molecule that would fit into the groove and stop the virus from binding to the cell. One day people may take such chemicals as part of their daily diet to prevent colds and other upper respiratory tract infections.

Methods of Self-Help

One of the most encouraging trends in American medicine is the desire of many people to improve their own health by simple changes in their daily habits. This seems to have affected the frequency of heart attacks dramatically. From having the second highest heart-attack rate in the Western world a generation ago, the United States has moved down to eighth on the list, and the situation is still improving. An analysis of why this has happened gives useful indications about the future of self-motivated preventive medicine.

Life-style changes, combined with improvements in medical care, seem to be responsible. For example, the full health implications of cigarette smoking have been investigated and the information made widely available. About one-third of all American cancer deaths (cancer of the lung, bladder or pancreas) are related to smoking. Although it takes ten years for an ex-smoker's risk to fall to that of a nonsmoker, the risk stops rising immediately after the smoker stops smoking.

Statisticians estimate that about one-third of heart attacks in persons under fifty years old are also caused by cigarette smoking. Less dramatic arterial disease (which accounts for many leg amputations) is also largely a smoker's problem.

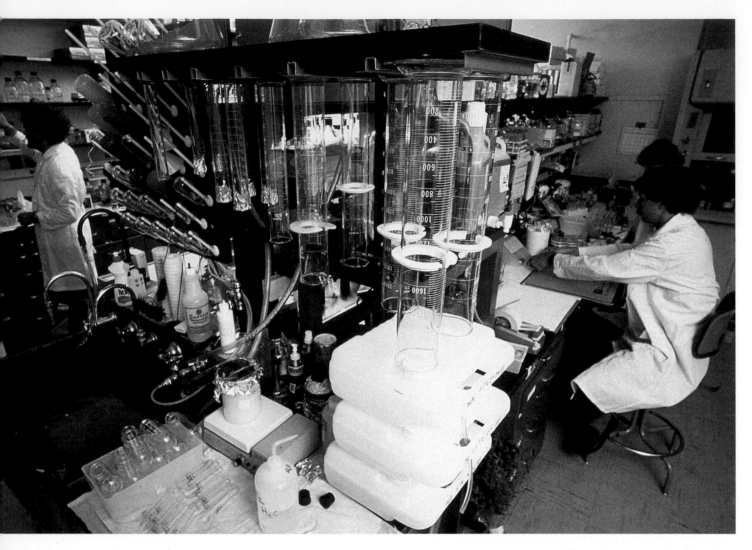

Molecular biologists are at the forefront of research into new drugs and vaccines. Together with genetic engineers, they are gradually accessing the blueprints that control normal and abnormal cellular activity and using this knowledge to produce new biologically active chemicals.

Many more women have begun to smoke since the 1950s, and the percentage of men and women who smoke is now about equal. As expected, the numbers of lung cancers in women has increased accordingly. One of the single most important factors in improving human health in the United States would be to eliminate cigarettes altogether.

Despite the implications of tobacco smoking on health, economic pressures from tobacco-growing states is intense. Tobacco is by far the most profitable legal crop per acre on suitable land, and many farmers' livelihoods depend on it. Subsidies to encourage them to grow alternative crops may be one solution, or perhaps countervailing economic pressure will build up. Many life insurance companies charge differential premiums, so that smokers must pay more than nonsmokers. The gradual spread of nonsmoking zones in public places may eventually inhibit new smokers, even if it does not have much effect on those who are already addicted to cigarette smoking.

The second most common cause of drug abuse is alcohol. Although the effects of alcohol on the liver have been known for years, it has only recently become clear that alcohol is involved in a further wide range of health problems.

Perhaps the most striking association is that high frequency of traumatic events that happen to individuals who have been drinking. Investigation of fatal traffic accidents indicated that in about one-third of them, at least one driver had been drinking. In fact, frequent involvement in traffic accidents, even minor ones, is now accepted as suggestive of alcohol abuse.

Many murders and violent assaults occur after drinking, such as a shooting following an argument in a bar. Indeed, the nickname "Saturday night special," applied by the police to inexpensive small-caliber handguns, reflects their frequent use on weekends in just this sort of barroom tragedy. Many suicides combine alcohol and drugs before killing themselves; this is especially true of people who are depressed by the effect of heavy drinking. Traffic accidents, murders and suicides are among the most common causes of death among young men. Thus there is a real opportunity for improvement in the health of the most productive element of society if their alcohol consumption could be diminished.

Alcohol presents a complex problem for the health planner. The effects of chronic alcohol abuse are largely dose-related and increase with the amount consumed, as do the ill effects of cigarette smoking. But the problems of alcohol do not need to be cumulative; a single acute episode of intoxication can cause death. Prohibition does not appear to work, so widespread education and advertising stressing the harmful effects of drunkenness, combined with improved medical and psychological techniques to help those who drink excessively, are probably the only ways to reduce alcohol-induced ill health.

Health Maintenance Organizations

A change in the philosophy of medical care is embodied in health maintenance schemes. Such prepaid health plans emphasize identify and reducing health risk factors before serious illness has developed. The organizations stress regular health

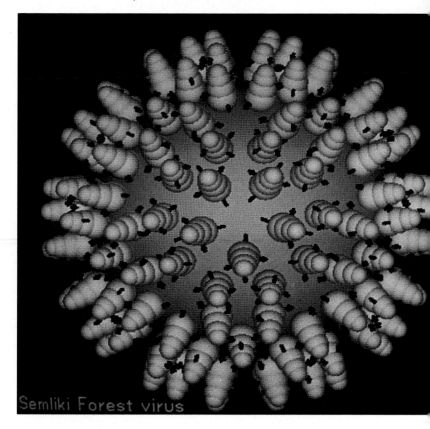

New insights into how molecules behave are possible with computer graphics. Sophisticated programs allow detailed three-dimensional models to be built up, such as this one of the Semliki Forest virus.

screening to identify problems early, and can also play a major role in reinforcing healthy behavior, such as stopping smoking and reducing alcohol consumption. And they have an expanding role to play because many studies have shown that it is almost always less expensive in the long run to prevent disease than to treat it on an individual basis. The cost of regular health visits and screening tests is far less than the ultimate cost of a major illness.

Help for Vascular Disease

Although preventive medicine will undoubtedly decrease the spread of disease, individuals will still grow old and develop the degenerative disorders that come with age. In particular, people will almost certainly continue to contract serious vascular disease, particularly thrombosis, in which a blood clot blocks a blood vessel. Striking advances have been made, and will continue to be made, in the treatment of age-related conditions.

Joseph Lister

Aseptic Operator

In hospitals today there is virtually no risk of successfully undergoing major surgery only to die afterward from infection of the surgical wound. Yet there was a time when up to half of all patients who underwent such operations did die for that reason. And that time was only about a hundred years ago. What turned wounds septic was then thought to be either the "spontaneous generation of germs" or some sort of oxidation process mediated by the oxygen in the air. That germs might actually travel in the air was first suggested in 1865 by the celebrated French scientist Louis Pasteur. But the fact that this proposition neatly combined the two supposed sources of sepsis, and provided a clue as to how sepsis might be avoided, was perceived by the English surgeon Joseph Lister.

Lister was born in April 1827 in Upton, Essex (in southern England), into the family of a well-known physicist and optical engineer. Educated at several private schools, he then attended University College, London, where he received a degree in 1852. He then went north, to Edinburgh, Scotland, where he became house surgeon and assistant to James Syme, whose daughter he married in 1856. Three years later, following the publication of a paper on "The Early Stages

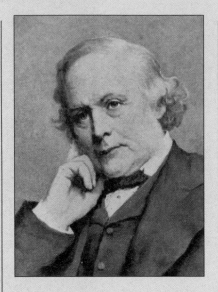

of Inflammation" — regarded by some as a classic, and certainly indicative of his open-minded approach to the problem of sepsis — Lister accepted the post of Professor of Surgery at the University of Glasgow.

In 1869 Lister succeeded his father-in-law as Professor of Clinical Surgery at Edinburgh University. After eight years there, he returned to London to take up a similar post at King's College. Between then and his retirement in 1896 he was knighted for his services to medicine (1883).

University College, London, has attached to it a great Hospital. Lister's early experience there with patients suffering from gangrene and pyemia (a type of blood

poisoning) influenced all his work thereafter. He was deeply frustrated by the way in which for many patients, even if surgery had been entirely successful, the efforts of the surgeons were being wasted by deaths from postoperative sepsis.

Pasteur's suggestion of airborne germs came at a time when Lister was in Glasgow. He immediately associated it with another contemporarily innovative discovery — that sewage used as fertilizer but treated first with carbolic acid (phenol) was disease-resistant. Lister began to use preparations of carbolic acid on patients with external wounds, as sprays in solution, as a paste with shellac in compresses, and so on. Within a couple of years he was able to reveal airily to an astounded British Medical Association that the Glasgow Royal Infirmary had, for months on end, remained clear of sepsis.

Such use of carbolic acid was not altogether satisfactory, however. Ten years of experimentation followed. After Robert Koch in Germany demonstrated the sterilizing properties of steam, Lister reorganized his methods so that all operating staff were obliged rigorously to "scrub up" before surgery and all instruments were sterilized.

Throughout history, inflicting pain by means of torture has been used to obtain confessions, as in the "dunking" of this unfortunate woman accused of being a witch. Physicians, on the other hand, have *constantly sought ways of relieving pain. Today there is a range of painkilling drugs, from analgesics such as aspirin to powerful sedatives such as morphine. But recent research into the properties of* *neurotransmitters, chemicals responsible for mediating painful stimuli to the brain, suggests that a major new painkiller without the addictive side effects of opiates might eventually become available.*

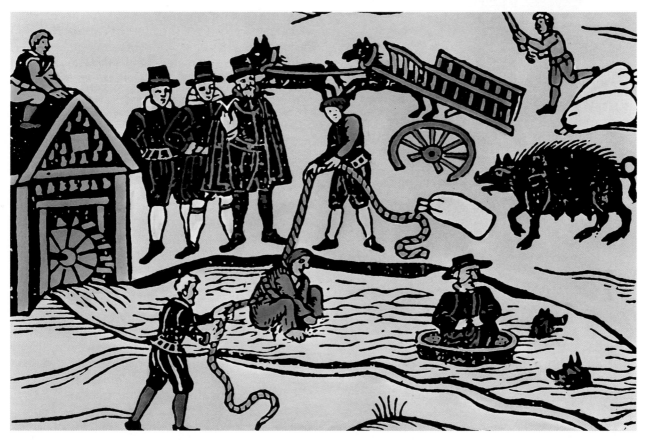

One promising development is the use of a protein called tissue plasminogen activator (tPa), which dissolves blood clots. Also an enzyme, tPa binds to clots and breaks them down, but it is limited in its effect and is unlikely therefore to cause severe internal bleeding (hemorrhage) as a side effect. The enzyme tPa is produced by genetic engineering and is just beginning to be used in clinical trials; the first results look promising.

If tPa is injected soon after heart attack symptoms begin, it frequently reopens a blocked blood vessel. If given soon enough after a clot forms, it could prevent the tissue death that follows a vascular occlusion (blockage). Also, because tPa has no anticoagulant effect, it can be safely injected into a muscle, and does not have to be injected directly into a vein. Ambulance attendants could administer it long before a patient reached the hospital — it might even be possible for the patient to self-administer it should the need arise.

Perhaps in the future we will all carry a phial of tPa and a syringe, and at the first symptom of a heart attack treat ourselves. Many other thrombotic events, such as blood clots in the lungs (pulmonary emboli), deep thrombosis in the veins of the legs, and even strokes may prove reversible with this enzyme.

An even simpler approach that may become standard practice is to take a small dose of aspirin every day. This idea was first recommended in the nineteen seventies, although attempts to prove its value have been confusing. The problem is to get enough people into a trial and then to ensure that they stick to the rules. The studies that have so far been completed show benefit for those who have already had a heart attack, and there is strong evidence that small doses of aspirin would prevent heart attacks from occuring. However, there is one major disadvantage in this preventive approach. The dose of aspirin that best inhibits clotting is

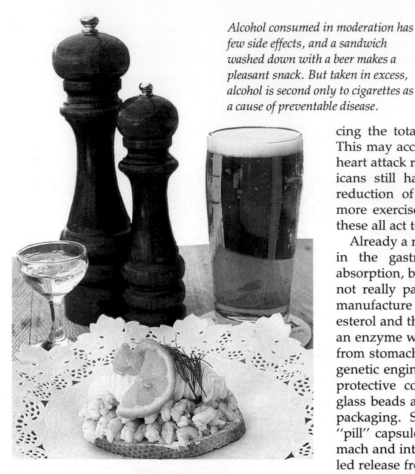

believed to be smaller than the dose taken for a headache — and it is important not to take too much: aspirin can cause irritation to and bleeding from the stomach lining.

A great deal of research has gone into trying to find out why the level of fat in the blood is related to the risk of having a heart attack, and how the amount of fat in the bloodstream is controlled. Fat can be deposited in artery walls, obstructing the vessels and making them more susceptible to being blocked by clots. The principal culprit is the fatty substance cholesterol.

Controlling cholesterol levels is complex. Part of the body's cholesterol comes from food, especially animal fats, and part is made in the liver. A critical control point is the mechanism that removes cholesterol from the blood and transports it to cells in the body where it is broken down. If there are too few receptors for cholesterol on the cells, then too much remains in the blood (because too little is removed). Excess cholesterol in the diet seems to reduce the number of receptors on the cell surface. The blood levels of cholesterol therefore remain high, and there is consequently more fat in the circulation to cause arterial disease.

The problem can be partly controlled by redu-

cing the total amount of cholesterol in the diet. This may account for the marked improvement in heart attack rates since the 1960s, but many Americans still have elevated cholesterol levels. The reduction of stress, less cigarette smoking and more exercise are probably also significant, since these all act to lower blood cholesterol levels.

Already a resin is in use which binds cholesterol in the gastrointestinal tract and prevents its absorption, but it has unpleasant side effects and is not really palatable. An alternative would be to manufacture an enzyme that breaks down cholesterol and that could be ingested with food. Such an enzyme would, of course, have to be protected from stomach acids and digestive juices, either by genetic engineering or packaging the enzyme in a protective coating. Although it sounds bizarre, glass beads are a possible solution to this type of packaging. Specially made glass can act like a "pill" capsule and carry compounds past the stomach and into the gastrointestinal tract. If controlled release from the beads can be achieved, it may prove to be a useful way of maintaining sustained release of enzymes before cholesterol can be absorbed through the wall of the gut.

Another possibility is a drug that would stimulate cells to produce more receptors for cholesterol-containing fats. More receptors would remove more fat, and lead to lower levels in the blood.

The Future of Brain Research

Knowledge of the brain and its chemistry is less highly developed than the understanding of most other organs. This is because of the brain's great complexity and the difficulty of untangling the intricate interconnections. It is probable, however, that brain research will be one of the next great growth areas in medicine.

For many years, little was known about the chemicals called neurotransmitters which help transmit signals from one nerve cell to another. Neurologists of today believe that neurotransmitters, and the receptors on nerve cells that bind them, are the key to understanding how the brain works and how some of its disorders may be successfully treated.

For example, schizophrenia and Parkinson's disease both seem to be related to the presence of

Diet, smoking, drugs and various environmental factors, ranging from pollutants to continuous loud noise, have been shown to be responsible for an increasing number of physical disorders and even to cause alterations in behavior, perhaps undermining mental health. The diagram illustrates some of these disorders and the major organs of the body affected by each category. Since these health hazards are largely preventable, medical research is being directed toward determining safe levels of potentially toxic substances, finding out how best to take precautionary measures, and introducing wider health education.

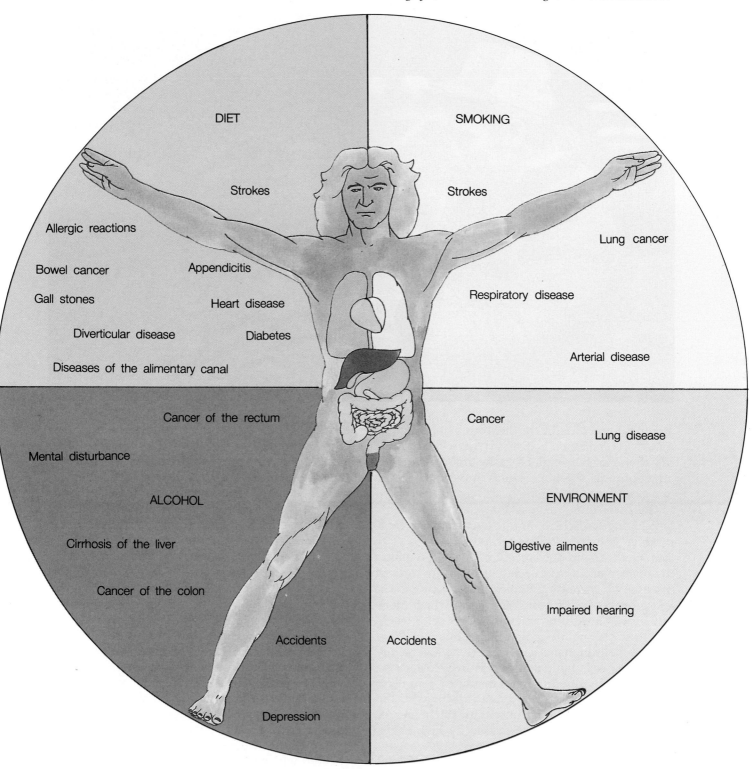

DIET

Strokes

Allergic reactions

Bowel cancer

Gall stones

Appendicitis

Heart disease

Diverticular disease

Diabetes

Diseases of the alimentary canal

SMOKING

Strokes

Lung cancer

Respiratory disease

Arterial disease

Cancer of the rectum

Mental disturbance

ALCOHOL

Cirrhosis of the liver

Cancer of the colon

Accidents

Depression

Cancer

Lung disease

ENVIRONMENT

Digestive ailments

Impaired hearing

Accidents

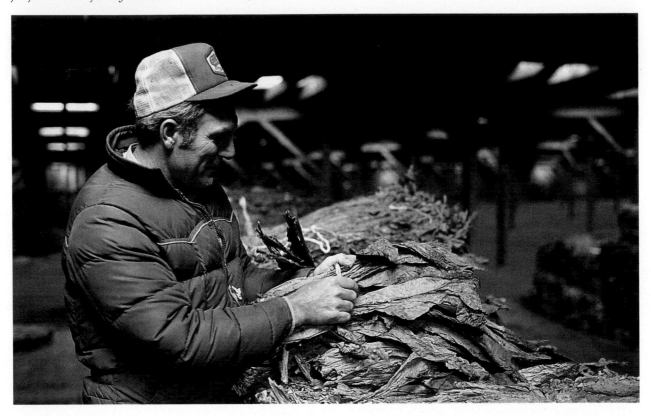

abnormal amounts of the neurotransmitter dopamine. In Parkinson's disease there is too little dopamine in some regions of the brain, whereas in schizophrenia the abnormality appears to be an excess of either dopamine or its receptor.

These insights suggest that one approach to developing antischizophrenic agents would be to produce better dopamine-receptor blockers or to find agents that reduce receptor levels. It is almost the reverse of the approach to preventing vascular diseases by increasing cholesterol receptors. The key probably lies in first discovering which chemical signals inside the cell control receptor levels, and then making drugs that mimic them.

Some neurotransmitters seem to be able to destroy nerve cells by making them overexcited. Release of large amounts of transmitter may occur during strokes, and some brain infections. If this proves to be a medically important phenomenon, then some of the damage caused by high neurotransmitter concentrations might be preventable.

Alzheimer's disease is a particularly distressing form of dementia leading to partial memory loss and disorientation. For many years it was thought to be a relatively rare condition that affected only the middle-aged, and was called pre-senile dementia. The dementia most common in the elderly was thought to be caused by inevitable aging changes in the brain itself. It is accepted that the process is the same in all age groups, and the Alzheimer's disease is, in fact, a common problem that increases with increasing age.

So what is happening to these people? Again, the first real clues are only just emerging and there are conflicting theories about where the cellular changes actually occur. But it does seem that a deficiency of the neurotransmitter called acetylcholine in at least one part of the brain is significant. The particular area of the brain most strongly implicated is so obscure that its name, *substantia innominata*, means "area with no name." It seems to be a critical relay station in maintaining attention. Perhaps it gives a sort of "wake up" signal without which the brain cannot form memories.

Remarkably, Renoir painted Gabrielle with Rose late in life when his hands were crippled with arthritis. Relief from the effects of the disorder may emerge from the discovery of a neurotransmitter in the brain called substance P, which appears to be involved in tissue response to injurous agents. If a way could be found to block its release, both the pain and swelling of arthritis might be avoided.

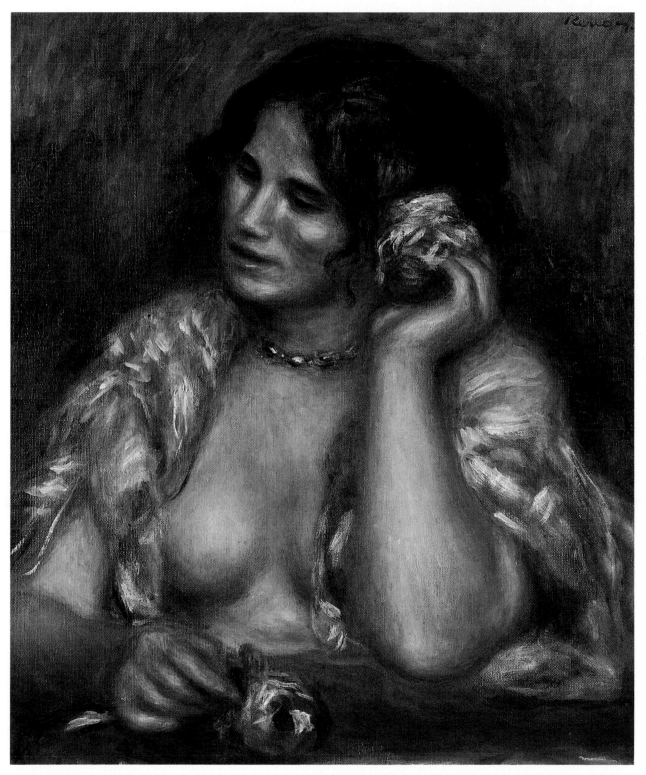

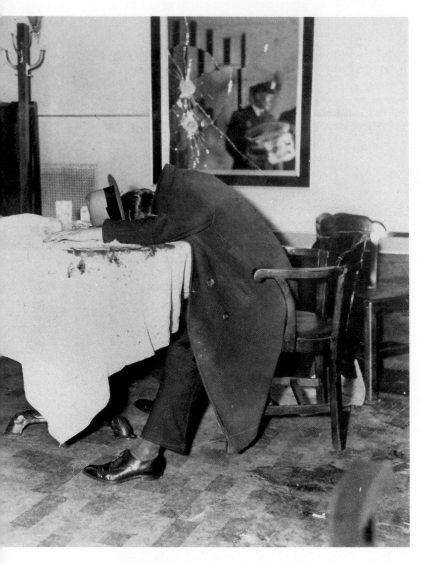

An infamous Prohibition bootlegger, "Dutch" Schultz lies slumped over a table after a shoot-out. Alcohol-induced crime is so common, police have named low-caliber handguns "Saturday night specials."

Acetylcholine is made in part from choline, which is a normal component of the diet. Attempts to improve intellectual function in people with early Alzheimer's disease by administering choline show promise. Certainly this will stimulate a massive effort by the drug industry to produce something to ameliorate the harmful effects of acetylcholine deficits.

Some neurotransmitters are so new that their effects are only just being uncovered. One of them, substance P, is involved in conveying pain sensation to the brain. Not only does it mediate transmission of painful stimuli, but it is also involved in the way in which animal tissues respond to many injurious agents. Inflammation, the painful swelling that accompanies injury, is partly caused by substance P released from the nerves supplying the injured site.

Two interesting possibilities present themselves. If substance P blockers can be made, they may be exceptionally useful in preventing pain signals during surgery or following major injuries. At the moment morphine is used widely because it affects both the initial perception of pain and the emotional response to it. But it carries the danger of addiction. By interfering with the release or movement of substance P, the possibility of a non-addictive major painkiller may be on the horizon.

Another possible use of inhibitors of substance P or its release from nerves could help to reduce inflammation. Arthritis is a common chronic ailment characterized by inflammation of the joints; already a little experimental evidence suggests that arthritis may be helped by agents that block the action of substance P.

Many neuropeptides, a class of biological molecules that include the natural painkillers enkephalins and endorphins, have been newly discovered. They have striking effects on nerve systems. Until recently scientists had no idea that they even existed, but now several forms have been identified and it is possible that a new pharmacology based on drugs that mimic or inhibit their action may be imminent. For example, neuropeptide-containing cells have been identified in the walls of the coronary arteries. They are thought to play a role in opening up or constricting these vessels in order to increase or decrease the flow of blood, depending on the heart's needs. Drugs with the same effect could possibly be used to increase blood flow to the heart muscle in people suffering from angina pectoris, a painful condition caused by a lack of oxygen in the heart muscle.

Neuropeptides may form a subtle transmitter system of communication between the nervous system and all the other cells in the body. An understanding of how they work may well give a better understanding of the links between emotion and disease.

Perhaps the most interesting development in brain research is that there seems to be developing a general agreement that many forms of mental illness are genuinely organic diseases; they appear to have specific biological or chemical causes. The extraordinary advances made by bioscientists in understanding the internal workings of the body's cells has set the stage for application of these concepts to the treatment of mental illness and to

Cardiac arrest is one of the most frequent reasons for emergency hospital admission, requiring the prompt and skilled action of a team of medical staff. Early clinical trials on a substance that "dissolves" blood clots, tissue plasminogen activator (tPa), may make such scenes comparatively rare. tPa is unusual in that, unlike other clot-breaking enzymes, it does not have an attendant risk of hemorrhage.

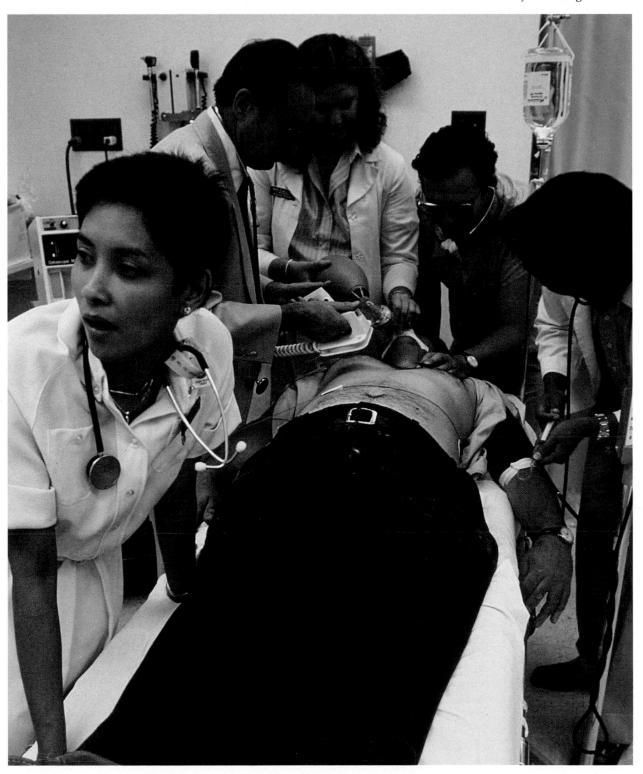

Norman E. Borlaug

Wheat for the Hungry World

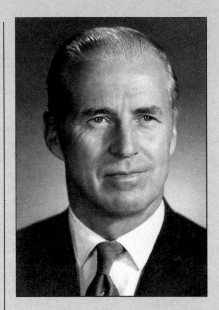

When the Spanish conquered Mexico in the 1520s they took to the New World supplies of wheat. As well as providing food, this grain was intended for planting; it was envisaged as a crop to replace the corn indigenous to Mexico. Four centuries later, some wheat is successfully grown in Mexico, but corn remains the country's staple food.

The reason for corn's supremacy is largely that the traditional varieties of wheat grow too tall and thin in the Mexican soil to provide economic yields. And because wheat is not particularly adaptable to variations in soil and climate, similar disappointments have occurred in many other parts of the world. Yet the nutritional value of wheat is such that, in the late 1950s and through the 1960s, the crop was proposed as the possible answer to the looming threat of Third World famine.

American plant pathologist Norman E. Borlaug was the "Apostle of Wheat." He has been the scientific leader of the "Green Revolution," and in 1970 was awarded the Nobel Peace Prize for his work on the genetic improvement of wheat varieties. In recent years he has lived and worked mainly in the vicinity of Mexico City.

Norman Ernest Borlaug was born near Cresco, Iowa, in March 1914, into an immigrant Norwegian farming family. He attended the University of Minnesota, where he received a degree in forestry in 1937 (and was also wrestling champion). After two years of forestry experience in Idaho and Massachusetts, and a year's research back at Minnesota University, he gained his doctorate in plant pathology.

In 1944, the Rockefeller Foundation set up a team to assist Mexican agriculture; Borlaug was an active member of that team. Initial problems included severe shortage of mechanized equipment, low soil fertility and a prevalence of plant diseases. Irrigation and the use of fertilizers on existing Mexican wheat varieties led only to even taller, even thinner wheat. The ears bore grain of little nutritional value on plants liable to keel over and die. The quest was evidently for new, sturdier, larger-headed varieties of the grain.

Some experimentation on new wheat varieties was begun in Japan in the 1940s. The agronomist Orville A. Vogel, working at Washington State University, used the Japanese results to derive a new dwarf variety named Gaines wheat. Borlaug thereupon used Gaines seeds to hybridize with Mexican varieties, breeding into the offspring the characteristics of adaptability to a variety of different environmental conditions. Eventually he produced a number of varieties that were both highly adaptable and high in yield. These varieties were usable in many parts of the world and — potentially at least — able to stave off world famine for some decades.

But Borlaug has not been content merely with supplying the means of nutrition to any country in need of help. He has also demanded a degree of commitment from the leaders of assistance-seeking nations — a commitment that has involved stability in government with a view to a complete agricultural program of maintenance and education.

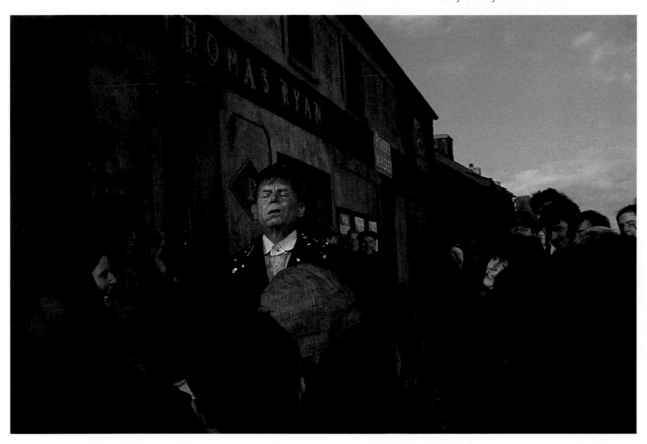

the possible prevention of premature aging-type degeneration in mental processes.

Who Pays?

As a result of scientific or behavioral advances, everyone can look forward to a better lifestyle and better medical care in the future. But who will pay, and what will the consequences be for Americans if that question remains unanswered? The fact is that the best medicine in the world is available in the United States. At a price.

When a graph of the mortality rate in the United States is drawn it shows two peaks: within a year of birth, and at about sixty-five to seventy years of age. A glib assumption is that neonatal death (death within a few weeks of birth) is largely caused by unavoidable circumstances. Genetic diseases, true accidents of nature, overwhelming infection of defenseless newborns all figure large in infant mortality statistics. But are these truly un-

avoidable? Could different ways of funding medicine and delivering medical care to people at risk reduce infant mortality?

Boston, Massachusetts, provides a sobering model. There are three world-famous medical schools in Boston, and some of the best hospitals in the world. Men and women trained in these great centers practice medicine throughout the Boston area. If ever there was a place where high medical standards are available to the whole community it is surely in Boston.

Yet in Boston, and probably everywhere else in the United States, infant mortality is high where parental income is low. Race, education and other factors do not seem to matter very much when the effects of income are factored out of the statistics. By implication, a child's health is related to the amount of money that is spent on it. So here is a major political question: should the Federal Government fund child health care for the poor? What

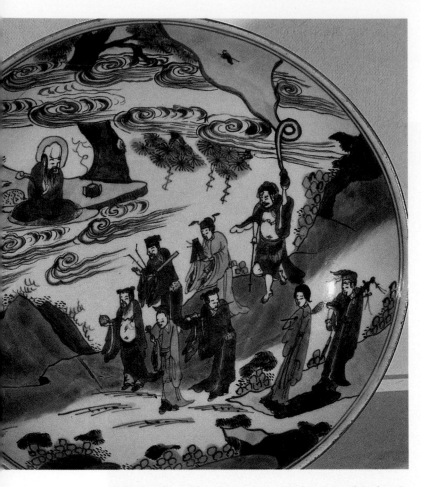

compulsory retirement laws enacted in earlier times. There may soon be an overwhelming demand for facilities that allow both part-time work and part-time physical recreation.

Can We Live Forever?

Can medicine achieve immortality, or at least allow people to live for two hundred, even three hundred, years? The answer is probably not, because all mammalian species studied seem to have a predetermined maximum life span, and, although no one knows why, for human beings this seems to be about one hundred and twenty years. In Western countries in which reliable records have been kept for centuries, there is no proof that anyone has lived past this age. Myths about phenomenally long-lived peasants in distant primitive parts of the world are probably just that: myths.

The longest-lived people in the world today are probably Scandinavians, some of whom have a life expectancy of just over eighty years. In Western countries, more people are living longer and approaching the theoretical limit, but if a life span of greater than one hundred and twenty years were possible it seems certain that a few people somewhere would have lived that long by now.

The scientific study of aging is called gerontology. By its very nature it is a difficult subject, because the length of its experiments must be measured in decades. A favorite explanation of why we gradually decline as we get older is that we accumulate tiny amounts of damage to our cells and connective tissue. The damage has to be repaired but eventually the capacity for repair is exhausted and further damage leads to death.

There is one theory that suggests oxygen may be responsible for much of the damage. Many of the body's defenses, especially those involving white blood cells (and thus by implication, the body's immune system), use a particularly active form of oxygen called a free radical. The oxygen radical destroys bacteria and harmful enzymes, but occasionally a little too much is made and normal tissue is damaged. One theory of aging holds that oxygen radical damage is the factor that makes us fall apart in the end. Since both vitamins C and E prevent oxygen free radical formation, they might contribute to slowing the aging process.

effect will recent cutbacks in federal health funds have? The importance of the Boston study is that, despite widely available advances in medicine, it is still money that determines who gets the best treatment.

Health costs will continue to be a political issue for the rest of this century and beyond. As the population ages, so the overall need for medical care increases. Aging carries an inevitable series of medical problems that can often be successfully treated — but the grim specter of bankruptcy is always present. So where will the limits of high-cost, high-tech medical care be set? It seems inevitable that, in the light of such questions, the large and politically sophisticated older population will press for increasing government health funding.

While the debate over medical economics continues, prospects for the aging population are improving. The most encouraging finding is that many people benefit from both physical and mental activity. Many of the supposedly inevitable consequences of aging can be prevented or slowed down — ''Do not stop'' is good advice. The healthy effects of continued activity have been recognized by many state legislatures by repealing the

Willow trees bend gracefully in the breeze in Constable's painting of a water meadow. Many natural products which folklore has maintained to be of medical value, particularly those obtained from

plants, are being investigated in the search for safe and effective new drugs. A few have yielded results — willow leaves and bark contain a substance similar to aspirin, for example.

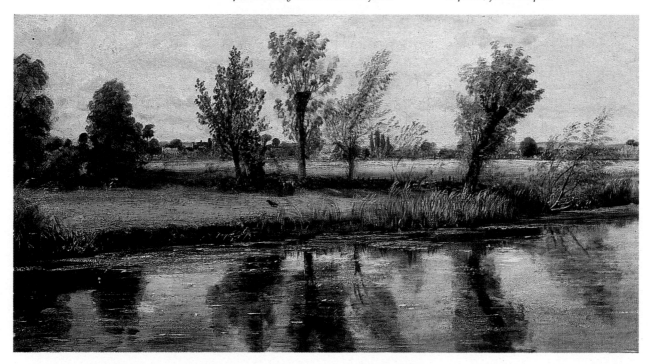

Most experiments to test various ways of extending life span use mice, because their normal span is only about two years. Even so, it takes many years to conduct a series of experiments. One of the earliest studies showed that mice raised and maintained on a calorie-restricted diet lived much longer than their siblings who had access to unlimited food. Over the years a number of natural products thought to prolong life (usually in folklore) appeared successful when tested in mice. But when the animals were carefully studied, in each case the treated animals ate and weighed far less than untreated animals.

The message from animal experiments is clear — measures that limit food intake and body weight regularly prolong life, and so far no other factor has proved to do this. Thus one formula for healthy living is probably to eat correctly and to avoid eating to excess.

It is unlikely that an immortality plant will ever be discovered, one whose consumption effectively slows aging and improves health. However, drug firms spend vast amounts searching for natural products that can yield drugs. Digitalis, the foxglove derivative, is used to treat heart failure, and its medical properties have been known for more than three hundred years. When penicillin and streptomycin were discovered to be products of common fungi, a vast search for similar organisms began. There were some successes. Many "folk medicines" were scrutinized to see if they really had any effect, and some did. South American Indians treated malaria with tree bark containing quinine, and willow leaves and bark contain an aspirinlike substance.

Occasionally something unexpected turns up. Vincristine and vinblastine are two powerful anticancer agents discovered during studies on extracts from the periwinkle plant, which folklore maintained was good for diabetes. In fact, the antidiabetic effect was not any better than drugs already available and the chances of finding a revolutionary new medicine from long-lost folk medicine are rapidly declining. Often the folk remedy works up to a point, but it is much less potent than something already on the market or it has more severe side effects. The new medicines of the twenty-first century are much more likely to come from the computer modelers and genetic engineers.

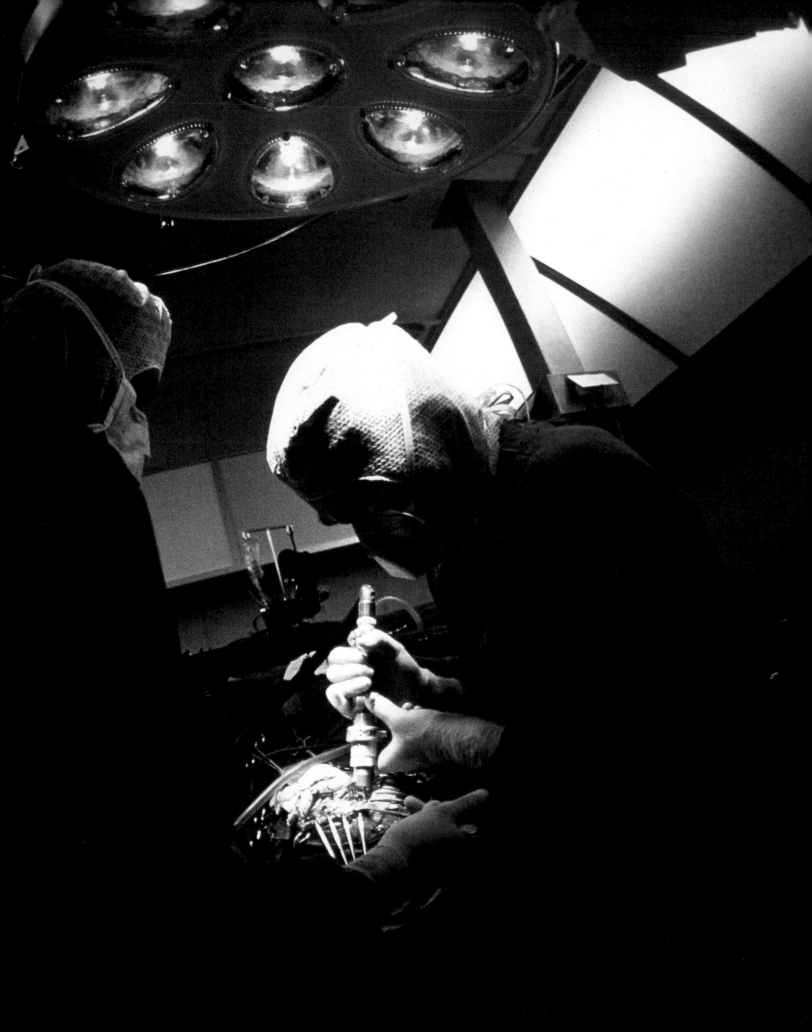

Chapter 3

The Bionic Body

The rise of modern surgery in the twentieth century has been marked by an extraordinary growth of technology and techniques. These have permitted the surgeon to explore virtually all portions of the human body, including spaces that seemed to be unapproachable to previous generations of surgeons, including the brain, heart and uterus. Advances in the basic understanding about body structure and function have increased the sphere within which the surgeon can operate. For example, such an expansion of knowledge concerning the heart has lead to a wide range of operations on damaged hearts, as well as to the actual replacement of the heart by another human heart and, most recently, by an artificial one. The same expansion of knowledge has also served to decrease the level of surgical activity, for it has enabled the prevention or treatment of illness with alternative techniques including chemotherapy and radiotherapy.

The recent discovery of drugs for treating stomach ulcers is an example. Each year, as many as three hundred partial gastrectomies were performed in large US city hospitals — now as few as five or six may be carried out. A medical breakthrough dramatically reduced the general surgeon's workload, even if, as some experts argue, the disease was already in decline.

Surgery — Future Prospects

General surgery may, in the future, have even fewer "customers" if Western nations heed the advice of nutritionists. Experts believe that a host of diseases of the alimentary canal could be almost wiped out if people followed a diet high in fiber and low in fat, salt and sugar. Many of these diseases do not exist in some of the developing countries of Africa, where the population eats a high-fiber diet. And there is little doubt that the incidence of diet-related disorders such as hemorrhoids, diverticular disease, cancer of the bowel, appendicitis and gallstones currently treated by

A surgeon uses a compressed air-powered drill to cut a hole through a skull in a life-saving operation. Despite spectacular advances in surgical techniques and equipment, most surgery will one day be regarded as a last resort. In an ideal future world it should become a rarity as breakthroughs are made in medicine and drug research. The major exceptions are transplant, replacement and orthopedic surgery, which can restore or repair damaged parts of the body.

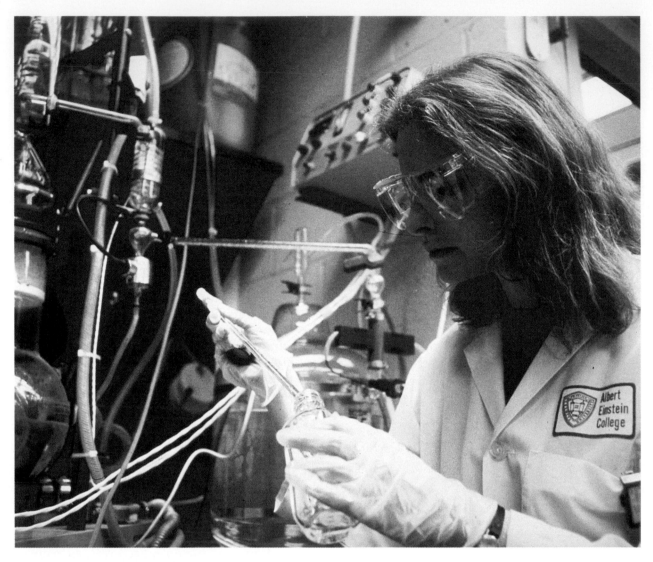

Developments at the forefront of medical research have resulted in a variety of ethical problems. For example, techniques such as chorionic villus sampling and amniocentesis, which provide samples of fetal tissue for analysis, can detect fetal abnormalities during pregnancy. But should a mother be allowed to terminate a pregnancy if it is known that her baby is abnormal?

surgery could be dramatically reduced if education about diet were successful.

Hope for Arthritis

A similar type of breakthrough is on the horizon in the field of orthopedics, much of which involves surgical treatment of bone disorders caused by degeneration or aging. Scientists have discovered that sufferers from osteoarthritis, a degenerative, often crippling disease of the joints, have defects in the antibodies of their immune system. Research into finding the cause is still in its infancy, but if it succeeds the workload of the orthopedist could be reduced by thirty or forty per cent.

Osteoarthritis is not just a result of old age. There are people more than a hundred years old who have no sign of this type of wear and tear in their joints, whereas many people around the age of sixty have extensive joint damage. Aging is thus not the only cause. Osteoarthritis was once

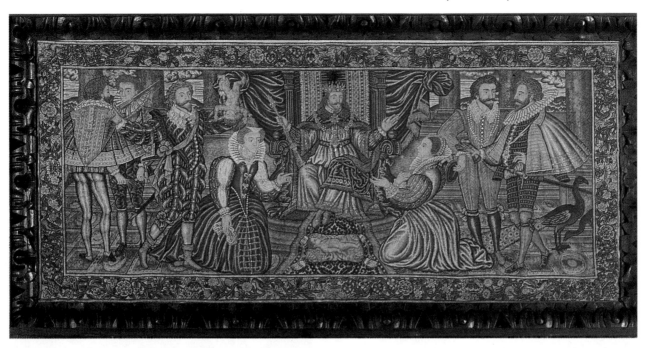

thought to be caused by a fault in the immune system, whereby the body failed to recognize its own tissues as self. But it now appears that osteoarthritis is not a true autoimmune disease — the sufferer's antibodies are not "eating" tissue — but something seems to go wrong with the normal chain reaction that is associated with functioning antibodies.

Under ordinary circumstances, a germ is marked out by an antibody as "foreign," rather as a tree may be marked with white paint when it is ready to be felled. The white paint does not harm the tree in itself, but distinguishes it from the others. In osteoarthritis it is as if, instead of the tree being marked carefully and with forethought, the white paint is being splattered around on all sorts of things so that when the body's immune system (the lumberjacks of the analogy) come into operation, all sorts of structures within the joint are indiscriminately destroyed.

Now that scientists have an idea of the cause of arthritis, they may be able to find a cure. And if they do, all the technological advances into hip replacement surgery, prosthetic knee joints, and a host of other orthopedic discoveries will become much less important and fade from surgical prac-

tice. In a similar way, years of experience and research into the surgery of tubercular joints and poliomyelitic limbs has become more or less irrelevant in the Western world with the conquest of tuberculosis and polio.

Genes and the Future

It seems likely that the cure for many disorders will come directly out of the information that scientists can now obtain from a person's genes. It is now known that many disorders have both an environmental and a genetic background. What else could explain the fact that, against unequivocal evidence that smoking leads to lung cancer, some people smoke eighty cigarettes a day and of this group some die of an unrelated condition in their seventies? It is thought to be because some people have a genetic predisposition toward contracting a certain disease.

At present, most medical research effort is directed toward identifying conditions that result in severe chronic disability or death in early life. As advances in the treatment of all diseases continue on a broad front, many conditions fatal even twenty years ago become treatable, with a good chance of a reasonable quality of life for the pa-

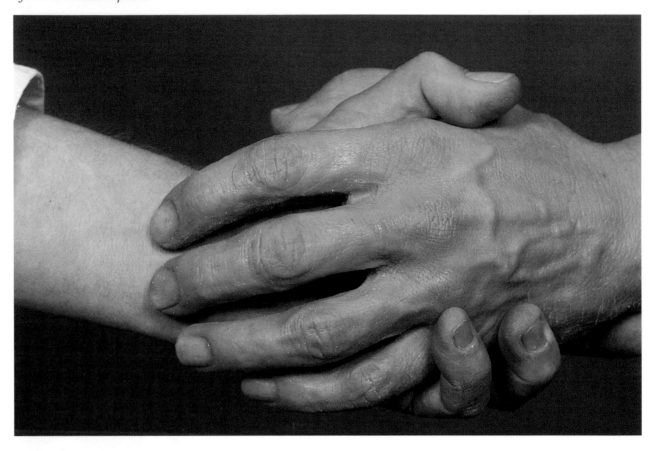

tumors from growing in the first place. One of the factors that sets a limit to the treatment of cancer with drugs is that the anticancer drugs are poisonous to bone marrow cells, the cells which manufacture most of the cells in the blood. Chemotherapy involving doses of drugs large enough to destroy all the cancer cells in the body may thus also wipe out the blood-forming cells. The result may be a fatal hemorrhage resulting from a lack of blood platelets, the cell fragments which help blood to clot. Alternatively, a potentially fatal infection may set in because there are not enough white blood cells remaining in the system to combat it effectively.

One method of overcoming this problem would be to remove some of the patient's own bone marrow before chemotherapy began. The cells could be stored deep-frozen in liquid nitrogen until treatment was completed, then the patient's own cells could be given back. New blood cells would then, in theory, be made and recovery would be complete. None of the "rejection" dangers associated with bone marrow transplants from another person would occur, and so it would seem to be a perfect solution.

Unfortunately, when this attractive approach was first tried it became clear that most people with cancers far enough advanced to require high doses of chemotherapy had cancer cells in their bone marrow as well. Although there were too few cells to see with a microscope, there were still enough to grow, spread and kill the recipient when reimplanted.

The existence of cancer cells in the bone marrow seemed to present an insurmountable barrier to treatment. But now there is new hope. A way had to be found to separate the normal cells from the cancer cells. This was difficult because there is no definite way of distinguishing between healthy and malignant bone marrow cells. The break-

One aim of medicine is to prevent or lessen the effects of disability. The range of artificial devices available to replace lost limbs and organs is large, as this diagram of "spare-part" man illustrates. Artificial limbs restore a large measure of normal functioning to patients. Their movements are powered by small electric motors which, in some cases, respond to electrical impulses from the muscles where the limb is attached. The problem with replacing internal organs is more difficult, because the body tends to reject any "foreign" invader. But prosthetic arteries made from plastic are widely used, and the world has already witnessed the first artificial heart transplants. Leading heart surgeons confidently expect the technology and surgical techniques to become refined over the next decade or so and replace conventional transplants. Looking even further ahead, there is the prospect that biologists will one day be able to grow replacement organs from cells taken from the patient's own body, thus overcoming any possibility of rejection.

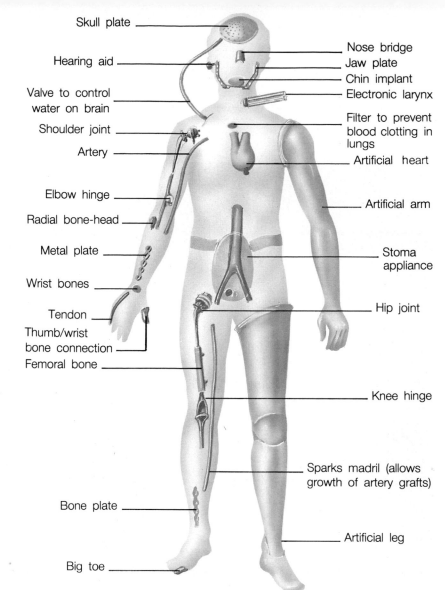

Skull plate

Hearing aid

Valve to control water on brain

Shoulder joint

Artery

Elbow hinge

Radial bone-head

Metal plate

Wrist bones

Tendon

Thumb/wrist bone connection

Femoral bone

Bone plate

Big toe

Nose bridge

Jaw plate

Chin implant

Electronic larynx

Filter to prevent blood clotting in lungs

Artificial heart

Artificial arm

Stoma appliance

Hip joint

Knee hinge

Sparks madril (allows growth of artery grafts)

Artificial leg

through came with the development of the mono-clonal antibody.

Monoclonal antibodies are defensive "particles" manufactured in the laboratory by the techniques of genetic engineering and can be produced in large quantities. Although it can be difficult to find exactly the right monoclonal, once found there is no danger of ever running out. Initially scientists hoped that it would be possible to produce mono-clonal antibodies that were totally specific for can-cer cells and could be used to kill cancer cells anywhere in the body. This has turned out to be a vain hope for most cancers, because there are no completely unique genetic "markers" for cancer cells. Most antibodies which were thought to be specific for cancerous cells react with other normal cells in the body. This limits their use as therapeu-tic agents because they damage normal cells as well as malignant ones. But there is a way out.

The normal cells in bone marrow do not react

with monoclonal antibodies that bind to cancer cells. As a result, monoclonal antibodies can be used to "purge" the bone marrow of malignant cells. Other approaches make use of the same basic phenomenon. In one approach, samples of the bone marrow are removed and allowed to react with the antibody. Then the cancer cells are either removed or killed. One ingenious method attaches the antibody to tiny iron-containing plastic spheres, so that when the antibody binds to a cancer cells it becomes coated with the iron pellets and can be removed with a magnet. Other approaches involve attaching a poison or toxin to kill the cancer cells. Either way the normal cells survive and can be reinjected after chemotherapy to eradicate cancer has been completed.

Environmental Trauma

If it became possible to detect and cure disease such as arthritis through gene screening, and to

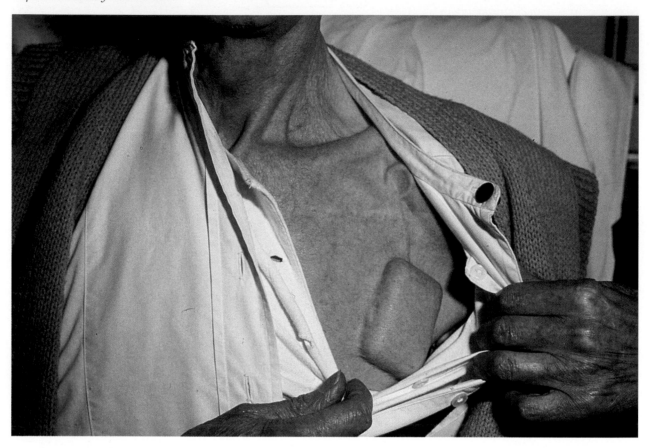

wipe out cancer by medication, environmental diseases would still remain and so constitute a large part of a surgeon's job. This includes the most shocking kind of environmental disorder — accidental trauma. There is no basic genetic predisposition toward crashing a car or falling out of a window (although these could be related to diseases such as schizophrenia which have a genetic element), so surgeons will probably always be faced with having to treat broken bones, cuts and multiple injuries.

Until now surgery has largely been concerned with taking things out of the body. The surgeon of the future, armed with more information about how our bodies heal and repair, will be able to use this knowledge to hasten the natural processes. At present it is possible to replace cartilage, but perhaps in the future it could be transplanted or — better still — induced to regrow of its own accord. Skin cells can already be grown in "cul-

tures" in the laboratory, and these cultured cells are being applied to areas of burns where they grow like a normal skin graft and cover the damaged area.

At present, only a single layer of cells can reliably be grown, on a collagen pad that prevents the graft from shrinking, but in future it may be possible for scientists to grow much more complicated structures. After all, a human baby begins life as a single cell and every cell in its body grows from that original one. Thus, in theory at least, it should be possible to grow full-thickness grafts of skin. Progress in this area is hindered by the fact that researchers do not have enough knowledge about the way in which cells differentiate into various types of tissue.

But this is too distant a possibility to speculate upon. It is more likely that advances in the field of prosthetic surgery, which is concerned with artificial replacements for joints, limbs and so on, will

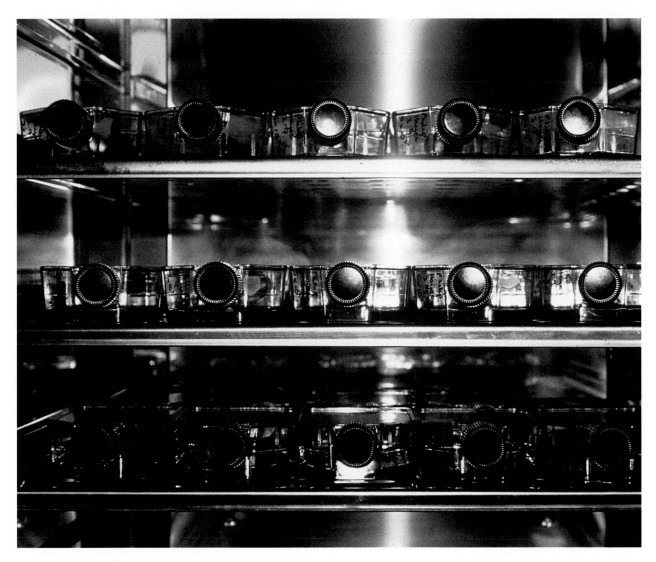

help people who have been involved in trauma. New materials are being pioneered that are inert in the body. A weight-bearing bone such as the femur (thighbone) can be replaced with a custom-built bone, and metal alloy hip and knee joints are common prostheses. In theory, there is no reason why, if necessary, all weight-bearing bones and joints should not be replaced with metal, plastic or ceramic "bones."

The risk of infection is crucial to the success of protheses, and this is the limiting factor in the development of a "bionic" arm. There is little possibility in the near future of attaching a complete mechanical forearm and hand onto existing nerves and structures in the stump, because even the smallest opening in the scar tissues of the stump would leave way for germs to enter and cause infection.

The other problem is that any nerve not connected to an "end organ" (because of injury or

Living human skin cells can be grown in flasks of enzyme solution, racked in a sterile temperature-controlled environment. The culture is made in two stages over a period of about three weeks. The cells can then be used as the basis of skin grafts to treat people with severe burns.

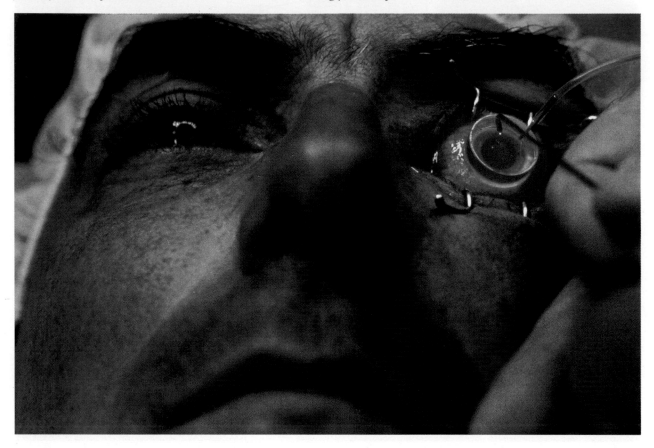

amputation) dies back along its length. It is not possible, therefore, to attach nerves onto a false arm and let the electrical currents — the nerve impulses — that moved the real arm do the same for the prosthesis. Instead, sensors are attached to muscles in the stump, so that when the muscle moves, an impulse can be relayed to the false arm and its hand. There remains considerable scope for improvement in the working of the mechanical hand following the advent of the computer microchip. It should be possible to program extremely complicated movements and patterns of movement into a fabricated hand, all of which could be initiated by a flutter of movement in the muscles serving the stump.

Even more incredibly, once scientists discover the key to cell differentiation, they could not only build complicated layers of skin, they might one day be able to program a body to rebuild a complete limb. Early in its life in the womb a human embryo has no legs at all. But within a few years of birth a human being has two powerful legs. It is quite possible to add to the body an amount of weight equivalent to that of a leg. The weight can be added either in fat, or in muscle through weight training. So why not grow a missing limb? Perhaps a limb bud could be transplanted to initiate the process. However good the materials for prostheses become, the ultimate goal must be to stop using prostheses altogether.

Replacing Nervous Tissue

One of the most difficult problems in medicine is that posed by damage to nerve cells. Unlike cells of the blood or the liver, for example, these cells do not divide in adults, and so they cannot increase in number to replace lost or damaged ones; once lost, they are lost forever. The problem is particularly acute in the brain itself. The brain's complex interconnections depend on the complete integrity of

A cataract in the eye's lens is one of
the most common causes of blindness.
In this microsurgical ophthalmic
technique, the lens is removed under
fluid pressure (A), before a new
artificial lens is inserted (B).

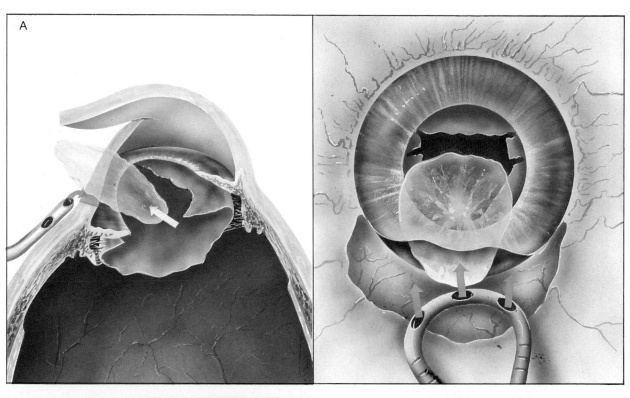

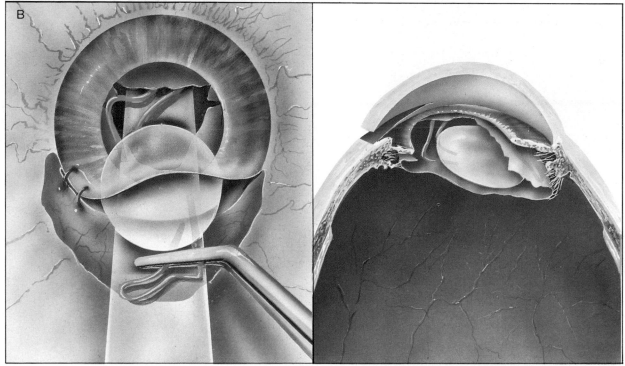

A brain-state analyzer (below) is used to monitor vital blood levels and to detect possible cerebral problems. Computer-assisted surgery will probably be increasingly used in the future.

Small stones formed in the kidney can cause agonizing pain when they pass into the ureter, and surgery may be required to remove them. A new technique (right) is safer, quicker and less invasive. The device directs a

focused wave of high-intensity sound at the stone, causing it to vibrate and break up, so that the pieces can be passed in the urine in the normal way. The equipment can easily be operated by nursing staff.

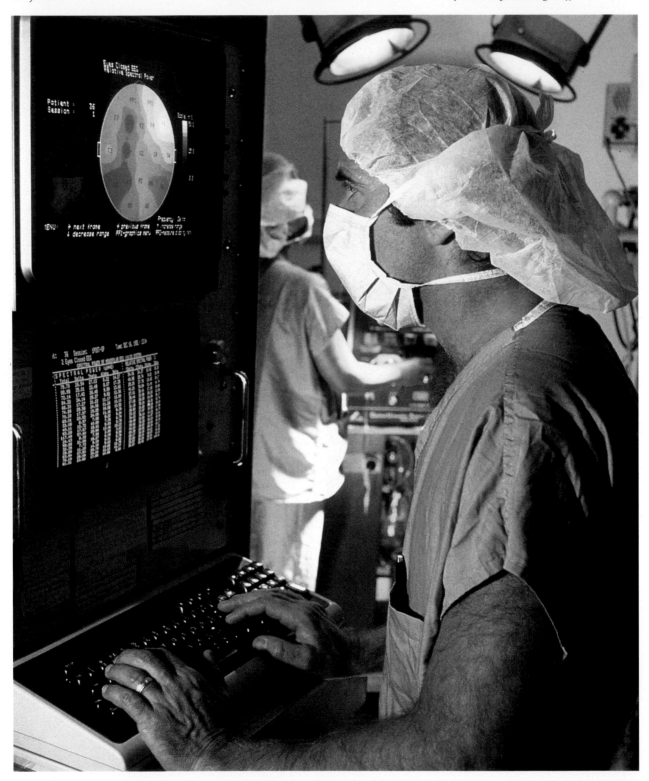

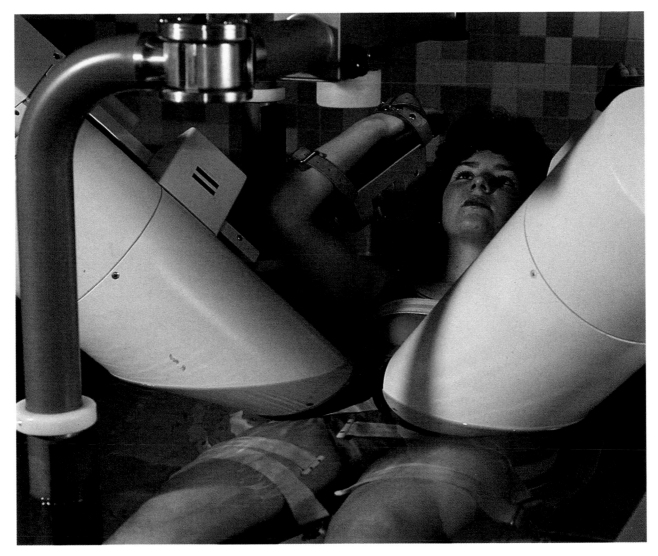

the whole network. If even a tiny junction point or relay station is damaged, a whole integrated function may disappear.

Two examples of this are Parkinson's disease and Alzheimer's syndrome. Both seem to result from damage to small collections of cells deep within the brain. In Parkinson's disease, cells that produce a neurotransmitter called dopamine are selectively lost and, as a result, motor function becomes disorganized. Sufferers have a characteristic shuffling walk and tremor of the hands. Although Parkinson's disease can be partially relieved by taking the drug L-dopa, which is converted into the missing neurotransmitter, this treatment is not completely successful. Alzheimer's syndrome may principally affect one small group of cells that produce a different transmitter called acetylcholine. The result is a catastrophic loss of memory.

The missing cells cannot be replaced naturally, because adult nerve cells do not divide and there is no way yet known to remove a few cells and move them to the damaged site. The cells just die. Nerve cells in adults are not flexible and, if moved, do not usually form new connections with surrounding cells. Only recently has it been discovered that fetal nerve cells are not so rigid. They normally grow as part of the expanding embryonic nervous system. They also put out branches to make junctions (synapses) with other nerve cells, often in distant parts of the brain.

Swedish scientists have discovered that brain cells in fetal rats can be successfully transplanted into damaged portions of adult rat brains. Although this shows only the barest glimmer of hope for the future, it does suggest an opening to be exploited. Indeed, the same Swedish group has already tried a similar experiment on humans. Cells from the adrenal gland, a rich source of neurotransmitter substances, were transplanted

*Central to the efficient running of a
hospital's health screening program,
the computer checks attendances and
organizes reminders to patients. This
increases the chances of detecting
disorders at an early stage.*

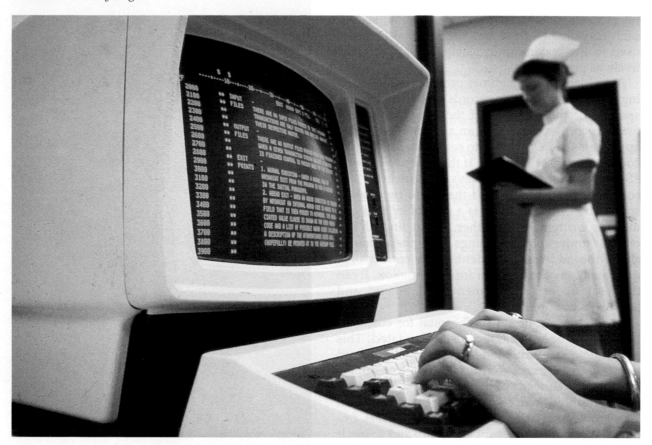

"conversation" with an expert (whether the expert is a computer or a consultant). Thus if a patient is to be quizzed for information by a computer, in order to diagnose any ailment he or she may be suffering from, it is obviously important to ask the correct follow-up questions. For instance, if the machine establishes that the patient is attending the clinic or the hospital because of pain, the patient naturally expects the immediate follow-up question or questions to concern the location of the pain (and not, say, eating habits). He or she would expect a physician to ask: "Where does it hurt?" If the "expert" does not follow up the appropriate question(s), the patient may rapidly lose confidence in the system.

Another implication concerns the sort of questions the computer "asks" the patient, usually displayed on a television-type screen. Impersonal communication is best avoided, and the more natural the dialogue, the more the patient feels at ease. Expert systems have been designed which explain their own procedure. This also enables the consultant to check the computer's reasoning for any particular patient so that, if necessary, the consultant can offer a second opinion. Of course, the human consultant can override the computer at any time and impose his or her own diagnosis. It is very unlikely that machines will ever completely take over control from human physicians in carrying out such tasks.

Once a diagnosis program has been written, the computer can begin to acquire data that should enable it to make better diagnosis. The knowledge a human consultant accumulates through experience is also often acquired over a long period that includes (possibly) only occasional or intermittent consultation with a patient suffering from a particular disorder, particularly if it is a rare one.

The computer collects its information systematically, and is even able to estimate the usefulness

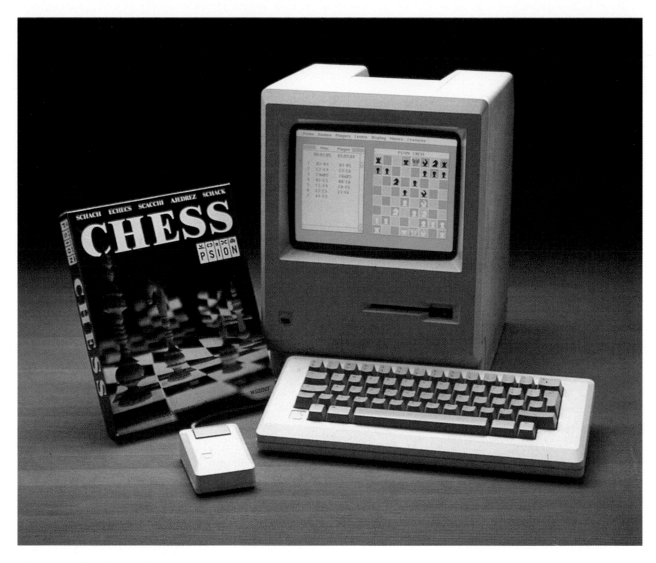

of particular data obtained from a patient for predicting the nature of a disorder. In this way, the accumulated data eventually enables the computer to improve its diagnosis. The consultant also has access to this improved diagnostic information and can therefore use it, should he choose, to increase his expert knowledge. If additional information becomes available (which was not included in the original expert system program), the program can be updated. Thus the role of computers in medical diagnosis is likely to be one of continual interaction between the machine and the expert.

Artificial Intelligence

Expert systems are one example of what has been called artificial intelligence. As the term suggests, it is concerned with getting computers to behave intelligently — to "think." Examples of attempts in this area include programming computers to play chess, backgammon or other board games, to

The chess-playing computer is one example of an attempt to simulate a human process — complex decision-making from a large number of possible alternatives.
Computerized models that bear close relationship to human functions are begining to provide a useful resource for medical research, diagnosis and treatment.

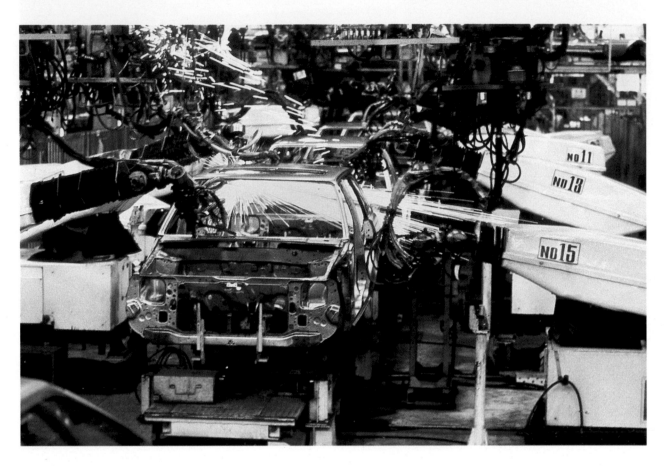

With humans needed to ensure only that everything runs smoothly, these cars are built almost entirely by robots. While it is unlikely that human patients will ever be operated on by unsupervised robot surgeons, the use of automated procedures in medicine is already evident. In the Soviet Union, one operation to correct nearsightedness (myopia) has become so popular that patients are passed along a line of surgeons who each perform a different stage of the delicate operation.

deal with natural language processing, and for controlling other machines in robotics.

Because computers operate so quickly, and can be made to have extremely large memories, it might seem that the way to teach a computer to play chess would be to write a program that generates all the possible legal moves and get the computer to choose the best one. But this is not how it is done. Just as an experienced chess player has a "game plan" which shapes up as the game proceeds, so the computer has too. The fact that both the machine's game and human players are governed by the same rules can be regarded as suggesting that a computer program may serve as a model of how a human player thinks. That is, the computer is effectively taught to play chess in the way a human does. So writing and then refining and improving programs that enable computers to play chess is thought to provide insights into the way most people play chess (or any similar game),

The fine network of blood vessels branching off the aorta into the kidney (below left) are revealed in this image displayed on the screen of an image-generating computer. A tiny throat microphone, a small control box and a set of ear tips comprise the Edinburgh Masker (below right), an ingenious electronic device that has proved to be of considerable benefit to people who stutter. The Edinburgh Masker works by generating a tone to prevent the wearer from hearing the sound of his or her own speech. The pitch of the tone alters with the variation in the wearer's own voice, thus encouraging normal intonation.

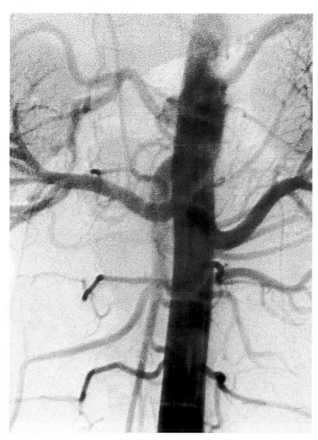

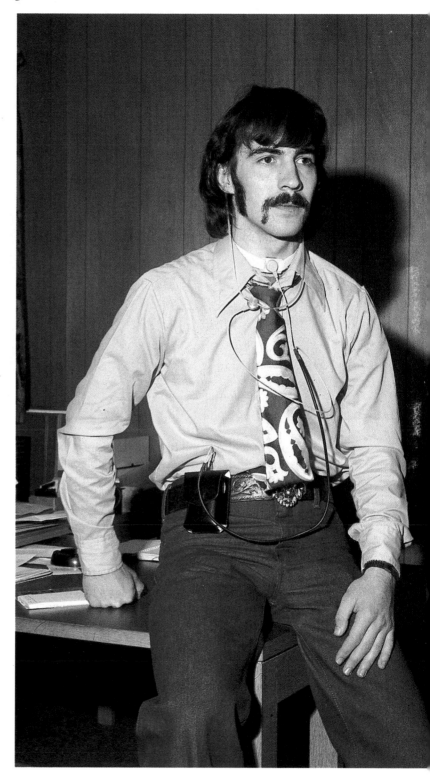

and possibly into the ways people solve other kinds of problems.

Similar principles apply to language. A translation computer does not generate every combination of words in its vocabulary and then choose the one most appropriate for some purpose. Instead, it generates only those that conform to the grammar (the "rules") of the language concerned. People who compile such programs are trying to learn more about how humans performs such tasks, with possible applications in the treatment of children and others who have difficulties in speaking and reading.

Computer-controlled robots may mimic other human functions and actions. They may have sensors — electronic "eyes" or ultrasonic "ears" — to locate objects, and complex circuits to generate patterns of electric currents to move mechanical arms and hands, analogous to the motor nerve impulses that control human muscular movement.

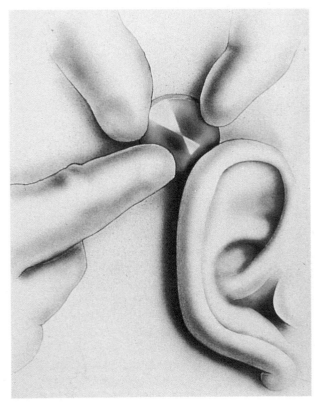

A similar computer-aided method makes use of the fact that certain atomic nuclei absorb electromagnetic radiation of particular frequencies and then resonate. The resonant frequencies can be detected and presented graphically on a computer screen. Called nuclear magnetic resonance (NMR) spectroscopy, or magnetic resonance imaging (MRI), the technique is specially effective at detecting tumors and other cancerous tissue. Like a CAT scan, it produces colored pictures of selected "slices" of internal organs. It is harmless and painless, and can be used to investigate soft tissues such as the brain and the lungs.

Aids for the Deaf

Hearing aids have long been available to help people who are partly deaf but whose hearing apparatus, within the middle ear and the inner ear, is basically intact. Conventional aids consist of a miniature microphone, amplifier and earpiece, which together amplify sound. Many can be tuned to match the frequency of the hearer's maximum sound sensitivity. Until recently, however, little could be done for people with damaged or malformed middle or inner ears. Then computers were enlisted to help.

In a person with normal hearing, sound funneled along the ear canal strikes the eardrum and makes the drum vibrate. These vibrations are passed on by three small bones in the middle ear to vibrate a membrane in the fluid-filled cochlea of the inner ear. Finally, it is the movement of this fluid that stimulates receptor cells to transmit a sequence of nerve signals along the auditory nerve to the brain, where they are analyzed and interpreted as sound.

In a person who is profoundly deaf, one or more of these middle or inner ear structures may be damaged. Often the inner ear lacks the mechanism that allows the fluid movements to generate nerve impulses. The auditory nerve, the connection with the brain, may be perfectly normal. So how can the auditory nerve be stimulated? One answer is to place an electrode close to it, send small electrical signals to the electrode, and in this way activate the auditory nerve to produce "sound sensations" in the brain.

Complete restoration of hearing is not possible

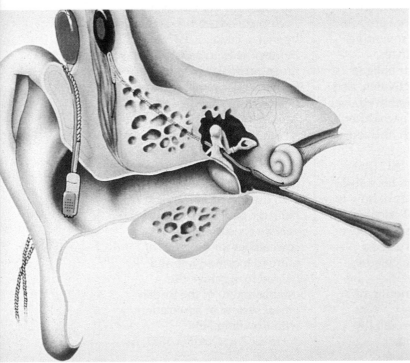

J. Von Neumann

Electronic Memories

Many surgical procedures in the modern operating theater are carried out with the aid of one or more computers. Presently, a computer may be used only to enhance the picture received on a screen monitoring an internal process of the patient, but in the future more use will be made of computers. Even by 1985 feasibility studies were taking place into the possibility of routine operations being undertaken by robot "surgeons." It was only in the mid-1940s, however, that the first fully electronic digital computer was constructed. Called the Electronic Numerical Integrator and Calculator (ENIAC for short), it relied on a considerable amount of manual operation involving pushing plugs into a plug-board and turning a number of programming switches in order to give instructions.

Within twelve months of ENIAC's completion in 1946, the concept of programming instructions, of storing programs, and of having access to that store in such a way that those programs could be changed if necessary had arrived. This gave the computer, in effect, a means of "learning." Computer theory was realized in practice in a machine called EDVAC (Electronic Discrete Variable Automatic Computer). The man

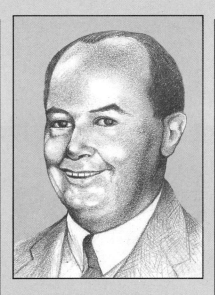

responsible for this innovation was the Hungarian-born American mathematician John Von Neumann.

Born in Budapest in December 1903, Von Neumann — whose Christian name at that time was Janos or Johann — was from the beginning exceptionally gifted in mathematics. He received a doctorate from the University of Budapest at the age of twenty, and became Assistant Professor at Hamburg University when he was twenty-six. In 1930 he emigrated to the United States and became Professor of Mathematical Physics at Princeton in 1933. In conjunction with that post he took on a Federal government consultancy with a brief involving the development of

the atomic and hydrogen bombs. He contracted cancer in 1956, and died in February of the following year.

Von Neumann has, with great truth, been described as "one of the last people able to span the fields of pure and applied mathematics." He was a mathematical theorist of genius. His combination of number theory and set theory, his work on groups, and his theory of rings of operators have all been called high points of twentieth-century math. He also obtained a degree in chemical engineering, was an accomplished physicist, and contributed to a classic work on the *Theory of Games and Economic Behavior* (1944).

From the late 1940s onward, Von Neumann's work was divided between physics and computer technology. The latter part of his creative output has strongly influenced the form of all subsequent digital computers, and was in great measure responsible for the "explosion" of interest in computers in the 1970s. But we may yet be even more grateful to John Von Neumann. His last publication — issued posthumously in 1966 — was an attempt to relate knowledge of the human nervous system to cybernetic theory so as to derive more sophisticated computer technology.

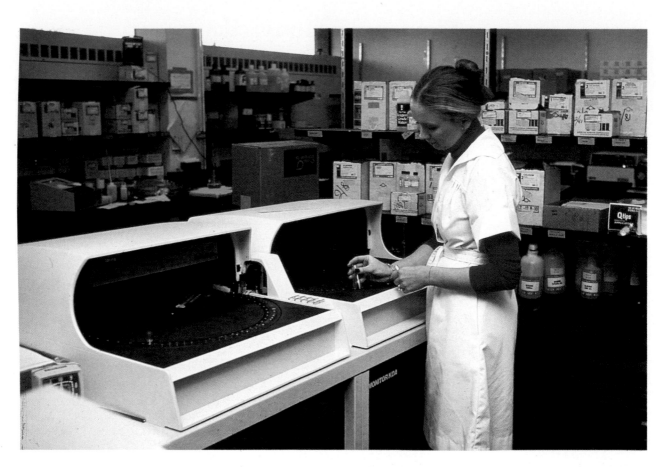

Physicians rely upon machines such as this computerized blood analyzer to obtain measurements of the concentrations of many blood constituents. Similar machines are used to analyse other body fluids, such as urine and cerebro-spinal fluid. The information is useful for disease detection and diagnosis.

by this method. What most deaf people miss acutely is the ability to communicate directly with other people. For this reason, scientists have concentrated on techniques that transmit some form of speech. The electrical implant makes only a small range of sound frequencies available to the patient. In one method, all the speech frequencies are compressed into the narrow band that the patient can hear so that much the same sort of total information is received as by people with normal hearing.

Another approach tries to select only certain types of information from the complete speech signal, and the best information to choose is that which cannot be obtained from other sources. These listeners are "totally" deaf, so the only information they do have is visual. They can learn to lip-read, but even then it is almost impossible for them to distinguish certain sounds visually — for example, the lips and teeth are in almost

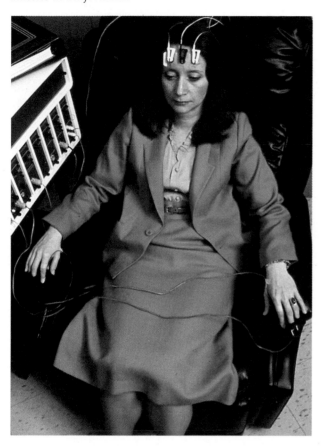

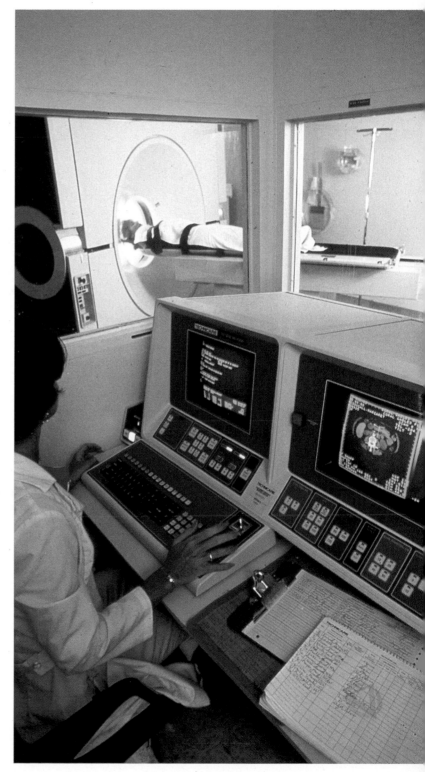

identical positions when pronoucing the "s" in "sit" and the "s" in "busy" or the "b" in "bat" and the "p" in "pat."

In each of these pairs of sounds, one sound involves vibration of the vocal cords (the "busy s" and "b"), whereas the other does not (the "sit s" and "p"). So that if the state of vibration of the speaker's vocal cords — detected by a microphone and interpreted by a computer — is the information passed to the deaf person via the implant electrode, he or she can distinguish between such sounds. It also helps in detecting subtle variations of speech intonation and therefore in distinguishing between questions and statements, and comments spoken genuinely and those spoken sarcastically. A group of researchers at University College, London, has tried this technique with some measure of success.

Computers are used in this research to analyze and process speech into a form that is suitable for

Technological advances may one day be able to release blind people from their prison of darkness. Utilizing sophisticated microelectronics, the design of one potential aid is based on the idea that the provision of sound information can partly compensate for blindness. By probing the environment with a beam of ultrasound, this device converts reflections from objects into audible sounds. The resulting sound codes the echo in three ways. The frequency (pitch) of the signal indicates the distance of the object, and the amplitude (volume) and clarity of the signal represent the size and texture of the object.

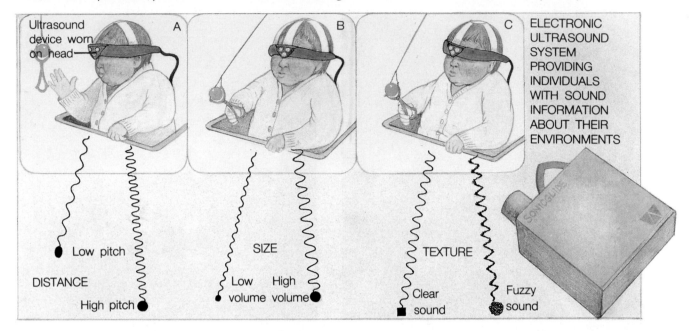

Ultrasound device worn on head

A B C

ELECTRONIC ULTRASOUND SYSTEM PROVIDING INDIVIDUALS WITH SOUND INFORMATION ABOUT THEIR ENVIRONMENTS

DISTANCE — Low pitch / High pitch

SIZE — Low volume / High volume

TEXTURE — Clear sound / Fuzzy sound

transmitting to the implanted electrode. They can either compress the frequency range, to feed in the whole sound signal, or extract the information indicating the rate of vibration of the speaker's vocal cords.

Computers have also been employed in research, to reproduce sounds in the same form in which they are heard by hearing-impaired people. People with normal hearing can assess these sounds and get the computer to modify them to deduce that, for example, additional pitch (frequency) information makes understanding easier. This might show a specialist what type of treatment would most benefit a particular patient. It is another example of simulation, this time to avoid costly and possibly ineffective treatment.

Aids for the Blind

The part of the brain concerned with processing visual signals is situated toward the back of the skull. If electrodes are inserted into this area and small electric currents passed between them, people so treated (even blind people) report seeing glowing points of light. Electrodes have been inserted in orientations that form a pattern which can represent all the positions of the dots in Braille. For instance, when the electrodes specifying the positions for a Braille letter "A" are activated, the person being stimulated can correctly report "seeing" a letter "A." A computer could scan a text and present the equivalent Braille signals, although the recipient could not decode them as quickly as the sounds used in auditory electrical stimulation.

In fact, reflected ultrasound signals acting somewhat like the echoes of sonar will probably prove to be a better aid for the blind. Most people with defective vision, or no vision at all, feel a greater need for the independence of being able to move around than for a method of reading, a need already supplied by talking books and other sound recordings. A portable loudspeaking computer carried by a blind person could analyze ultrasonic echoes and give the angle and direction to nearby walls or other obstacles. In one refinement of this idea, changes in the pitch (frequency), volume (amplitude) and quality of the echoes — reduced to audible frequencies — can be correlated with the range, size and texture of an object, respectively. Another prototype system, suited to workplaces such as offices, uses a high-frequency radio signal which is "piped" along a cable encircling the area. The blind person carries a receiver or detector, which inductively picks up the signal.

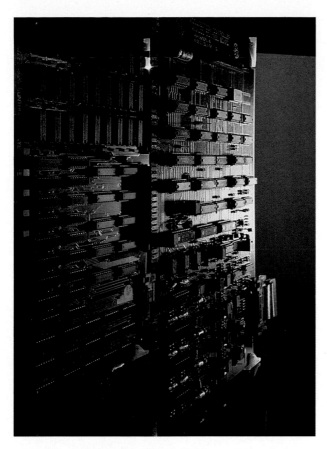

Many of the sophisticated devices of advantage to modern medicine require the power of a mainframe computer to operate them. Thanks to modern microminiaturization their thousands of electronic circuits can be housed in a medium-sized closet (above). Miniaturization can provide other benefits, too. Unlike a conventional wristwatch, this wonder of modern microelectronics (right) has neither hands nor digits. Designed for the blind and weak-sighted, it has a synthesized voice which literally tells the time at the touch of a button.

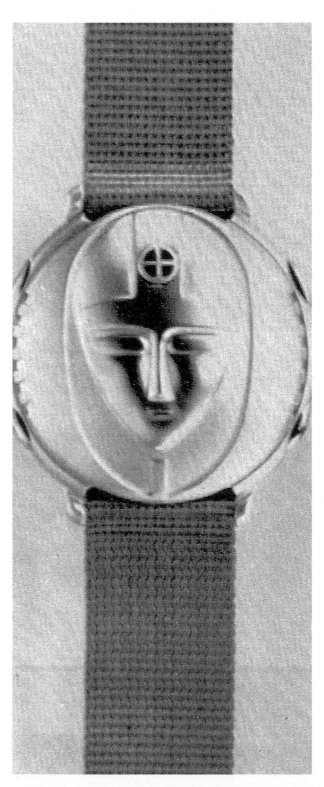

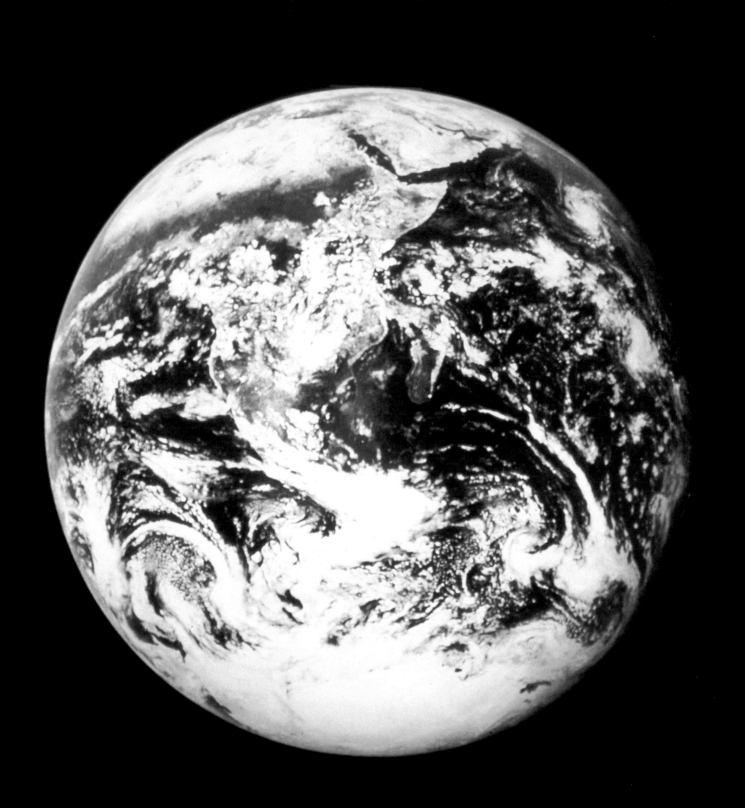

Chapter 5

The Body and the Environment

People often say that "the earth provides exactly the right conditions for life." The physical and chemical environments of the world are ideally suited to the organisms — including *Homo sapiens* — that populate the planet. The upper atmosphere shields delicate living cells from most of the sun's lethal ultraviolet radiation and the bombardment of cosmic particles. Sunlight filters through the atmosphere at the required levels to bring about photosynthesis in green plants. Apart from a few microorganisms, all creatures either eat plants or eat animals that feed off plants. In this way, sunlight ultimately provides the energy to drive all life processes.

On earth, the temperatures, except for those at the poles, are generally those at which biochemical reactions run efficiently. Water covers the planet in abundance — and the chemicals of life exist in a watery solution. The basic energy-manipulating and transferring pathways used by plants and animals require oxygen, and oxygen makes up approximately one-fifth of the atmosphere (most of the remainder is nitrogen). It might seem amazing, at first sight, that these conditions should combine to form the perfect environment for life.

But this logic is, of course, back to front. The argument here is similar to saying that the Mississippi is an amazing river because it just happens to flow through many major towns in the southern United States. The river was there first, and the towns grew up on its banks. Similarly, the earth was here first, and life evolved and adapted to fit in with the conditions that the planet provided.

What have been the "design constraints" on structure and function as the human body has evolved? If environmental conditions alter significantly, will human health suffer? Health need not necessarily suffer in terms of worsening states of disease, but could be affected by physical and chemical shocks to the system resulting from what the biologists have come to call "maladaptation to the non-living environment."

The Earth is humankind's birthplace — its health and ours are inextricably linked together. Earth, air, water and fire were the four elements of ancient philosophy. And humankind needs all of them. The human body is comprised of about sixty-five per cent water, because water is essential for most of the chemical processes that fuel our cells. Air, or more precisely the oxygen it contains, is equally vital for life. From the Earth humankind obtains food and essential trace chemicals. Without the fire of the Sun, life on Earth would be impossible.

103

What happens to the human body in the microgravity conditions in Earth orbit? Evidence from experiments on board the Space Shuttle, and from the Soviet Union's Soyuz space station program, reveals a certain deterioration of muscle fiber and a deficiency in bone-building. Any ill-effects caused by the space environment must be fully investigated before humans can make long-term space missions.

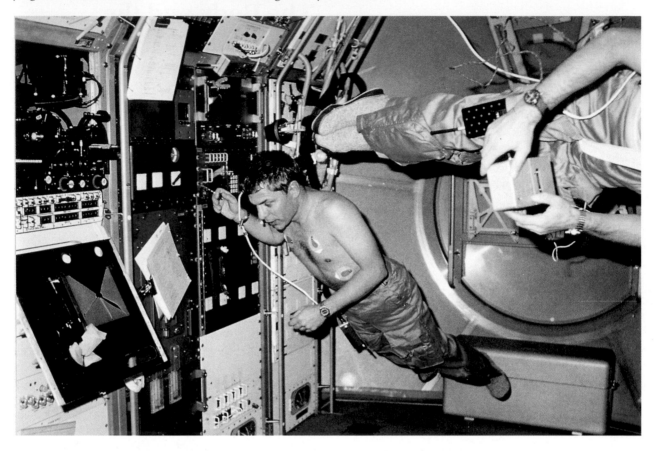

In less scientific language the "naked ape" — to use British anthropologist Desmond Morris's term for humankind — should stay with the conditions in which he evolved. The human body, unaided, should not go where it was not designed to go. In order to preserve human health, therefore, people presumably need to conserve the physical and chemical environment into which the human evolved. If they wish to explore new domains, they will have to take those "normal" conditions with them. Either that, or they must usurp natural evolutionary forces and adapt themselves, via biotechnology and redirected medical science, to any new environment they create or explore.

Taking the Weight off One's Feet

Weightlessness might sound like fun — but it can damage your health. Astronauts on long-term missions aboard Skylab and Salyut space stations have been studied intensively for the effects of zero gravity. Initially it was found that their bones became "demineralized" — that is, there was a loss of calcium and other minerals from the bone tissue. The bones became weaker. Weightlessness also altered the normal distribution of body fluids. Blood and other fluids, normally pulled down by gravity, pooled in the faces and upper bodies of astronauts, leaving their legs thin and spindly. Muscles also lost their strength through lack of exercise, so that when the astronauts returned to normal gravity at the earth's surface they had difficulty standing and walking.

These physical effects of weightlessness can be counteracted by training programs carried out regularly while the body is in zero gravity. Such exercises are now obligatory for Space Shuttle crews. The experience emphasizes the need for some form of artificial gravity in future long-term spaceships or colonies. Planners had always reckoned that gravity would be required in such condi-

A NASA concept of an Earth-orbit space station for the next century is illustrated in this artist's impression. The station would be constructed on a rotating wheel principle — the rotation around a central axis creates a centrifugal force that acts as artificial gravity. Construction in space should prove relatively simple; the station could be built of lightweight aluminum units. The stresses that such a building would experience would be far less than for a similar structure on Earth. The first such stations will probably be scientific observation posts, manned on a rota basis in a similar way to ocean-based oil rigs today.

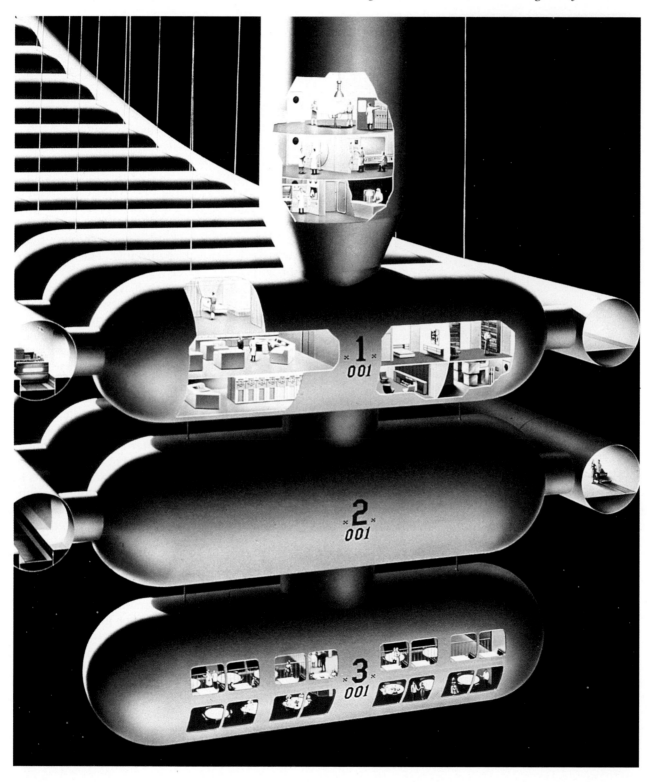

The ocean is an environment as hostile as space, and one almost equally unexplored. Divers can work to depths of about one hundred feet, but below this the cold and intense pressures of the ocean depths can be explored only in strengthened diving bells and bathyscaphs. It is likely to take many decades of continuing research before human beings will be ready and able to colonize this most daunting of environments.

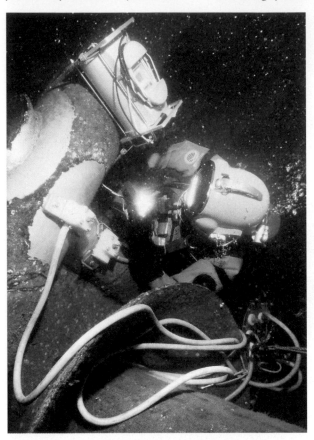

pressure to normal allows the nitrogen to come out of solution too quickly, forming bubbles in the bloodstream. This painful — formerly often lethal — condition is termed "the bends," decompression sickness or caisson disease.

To Boldly Go. . . .

Creation of "mini-environments" suitable for human life, such as the inside of a spacecraft, or a bathysphere, or an Arctic base, allows people to travel to, remain in and study previously inhospitable regions. For example, the American scientific station at the South Pole, on the great frozen continent of Antarctica, has almost every home comfort: a store, movie theater, canteen, gym, sauna, bar and private bedrooms. The accommodation is housed under a geodesic dome sited a hundred yards from the true South Pole, where outside temperatures can fall as low as −115°F.

Semi-permanent mini-environments such as the polar base have allowed researchers to contribute enormously to scientific knowledge. But so far people have really made only temporary trips, taking everything they need with them. A submarine carries its own supplies of food and drink; when these run out it must be restocked. Even chemically-produced oxygen — made, for example, by the electrolysis of water — needs continual raw materials (in this case water) and an energy source (electricity) to liberate it. If humankind is to progress to more grandiose projects, such as deep-space travel or permanent undersea colonies, there has to be more research into novel living environments. Scientists must create conditions for human life in the most economical way, making the very best use of the resources available.

For example, interstellar space journeys will take many years. *Daedalus* is a starship designed by the British Interplanetary Society for just such travel. Using a nuclear fusion reactor — which will probably not be developed for many decades yet — this spacecraft might travel at something like one-tenth of the speed of light. Even at this high velocity it would take forty-three years to reach Proxima Centauri, the nearest star to Earth after the Sun. This would require a truly vast supply of food, drink, fuel for warmth, and oxygen to support the human crew.

tions, and could be provided by centrifugal force through rotation of a wheel-shaped structure. It was assumed that since humans had evolved in a gravitational field, they would require one in the future. However, it was only when astronauts actually lived under weightless conditions for weeks at a time that the effects on the human body and their implications for health became clear.

Air pressure places similar limitations on human adaptability. The gases dissolved in blood (mainly oxygen and carbon dioxide) are at normal atmospheric pressure. Beneath the surface of the sea, the ambient pressure rises tremendously. After deep-sea divers have spent some hours at these vastly increased pressures, they have to be brought back to surface conditions very, very slowly, usually by a series of decompressions in a special chamber. This is because the extra pressure of the depths has forced higher levels of dissolved gases, especially nitrogen, into their blood. Sudden return of the

Arthur C. Clarke

Living in Space

"Space: the final frontier. . ." For thousands of years, until 1957, that was true. But since a few decades before, and for the decades since, that frontier has not seemed so unapproachable. Scientists now know much about survival in space — the sort of environment required, the equipment necessary, and above all, the continual monitoring of the biological processes of astronauts, right down to the measurement of the psychological stress. Initially, science fiction forewarned us of what to expect; then the technology of science became familar through the combination of space fiction television programs (some with more elements of fantasy intermixed), and of the actual broadcast relays of events genuinely occurring in space.

Basic to both the literary world of science fiction and to the world of space on television are the few scientists at the forefont of the relevant disciplines who are, in addition, excellent communicators. One such — a science fiction writer whose work is generally acknowledged to comprise far more science than fiction — is Arthur C. Clarke, the inventor of the notion of geosynchronous orbits for satellites which can be used for communications.

Arthur Charles Clarke was

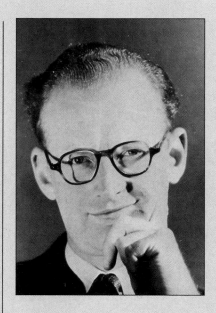

born in December 1917 in Minehead, in south-western England. After boarding school he attended King's College, London, until his academic progress was interrupted by World War II. During the war he was one of the very first radar instructors, a Technical Officer on the first Ground Controlled Approach radar system, with the rank of Flight-Lieutenant. It was at the end of the war that he made his suggestion concerning communications satellites. Returning to university he finally gained an honors degree in physics and mathematics in 1948.

Writing then claimed most of his time. He edited several books on astronomical themes,

and he wrote novels and short stories that became highly popular. By the later 1960s his renown was such that CBS Television invited him to take on the commentary for the space flights of Apollo 11, 12 and 15. In the minds of many millions, therefore, Clarke became closely associated with the "great leap for mankind" when, inside a matter of just forty-two months between July 1969 and December 1972, a total of twelve men had stood upon the surface of the Moon.

The 1970s thus saw many millennia of speculation resolved into knowledge; science fiction had become fact. But for that to have happened at all required two combinatory factors: scientific discovery had to have had the imagination to be able to comprehend all that might be necessary in so great an adventure — and to be able to furnish it; and popular interest had already to be at a high level so as fully to support national efforts to maintain a space program. On both accounts Arthur C. Clarke made a significant contribution.

Based now for more than twenty years in Sri Lanka, where he has a small research laboratory, Clarke claims to have retired from writing. His past work, however, continually earns him new honors and awards.

All animals need oxygen to release energy for cell metabolism. Fish draw in the oxygen dissolved in water through their gills. The semiporous membrane around this rabbit's cage performs exactly the same function.

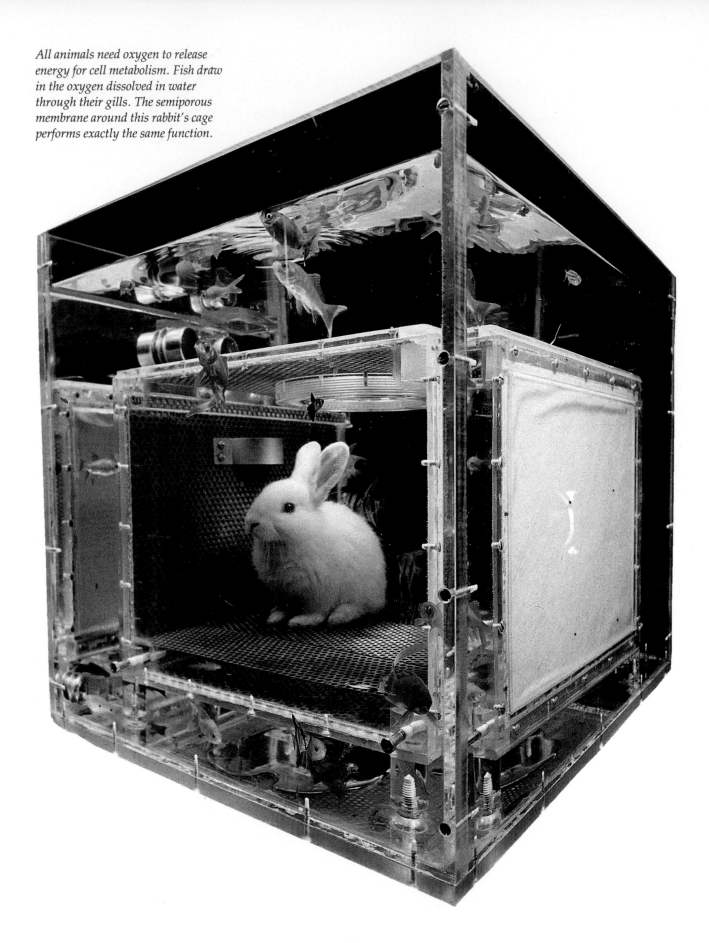

The nature of the provisions taken on any such journey has provoked much discussion. Should the food be preserved or fresh? Theoretically it is possible to live on preserved food, but fresh ingredients would do wonders for morale. What about a small fruit orchard and vegetable patch? Fiber-rich plant food is necessary for healthy digestive functioning, and current evidence suggests that constipation, cancer of the colon and several other intestinal disorders are more likely in those who eat too little fiber. This makes the "total meal in a pill" an unlikely eventuality.

Perhaps the starship should be stocked, as were sailing ships of old, with pigs, lambs and turtles. But modern nutritionists say that most people in the West consume far too much meat — so perhaps meat should be left out. If livestock were considered essential, goats and rabbits would make a good choice because they can eat a large range of otherwise wasted plant matter, and they are highly energy-efficient at converting it into meat. The animals could be allowed to breed, to maintain continual stocks of meat.

A totally different solution would be to adapt the crew to space, rather than vice versa. Cryobiologists, who study the effects of ultra-low temperatures on living matter, are researching ways of preserving organisms in suspended animation at very low temperatures. All biochemical reactions would proceed infinitely slowly or stop altogether, so that no resources would be required. At the end of the journey, thawing would result in reactivation, as if no time had passed.

This entire cycle is possible at present only with small, simple organisms such as yeasts and algae, and with sperms, eggs and embryos. But it may eventually be applicable to mature humans. Some type of cryopreservative would be perfused into the body, to minimize the damage to membranes and other cellular structures that occurs during the thawing cycle. The body temperature would be quickly reduced to minus 255°F, perhaps even lower. So frozen, the crew could travel through deep space with no aging or boredom.

Fish Out of Water

Artificially reproducing normal living conditions for the inhospitable undersea environment, for

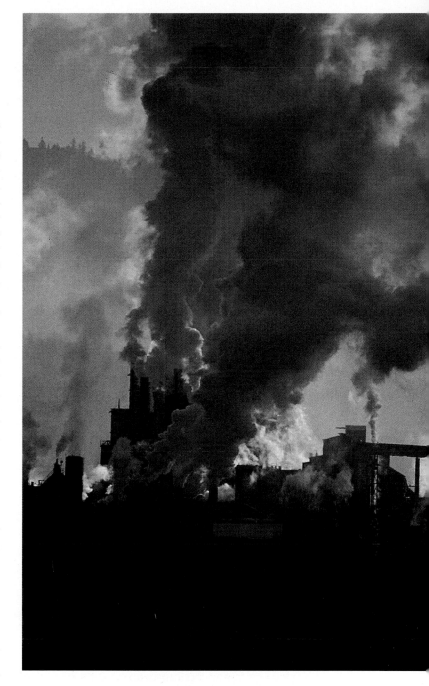

Industry and agriculture have had a major effect on the environment, often for the worse. Smogs caused by factory smoke and automobile exhaust are a major factor in respiratory diseases. Toxic chemicals discharged into the air, and into seas and rivers, have been implicated in causing certain cancers. In recent years people have come to realize that a well-managed healthy environment makes for a healthy life for everyone.

Water is an essential chemical for life but, as a carrier for disease organisms and toxic chemicals, it can also become an agent of death. At Minamata, in Japan, in the 1950s and 1960s, the pollution of a bay had tragic consequences. Inorganic mercury, discharged by a local factory, was converted into organic mercury by marine algae. This was eaten by crustaceans and small fish, and deadly concentrations built up along the food chain, as the diagram shows. The local diet was based on fish, and the toxic levels of mercury resulted in a dramatic rise in brain damage and birth defects among the children of the local population.

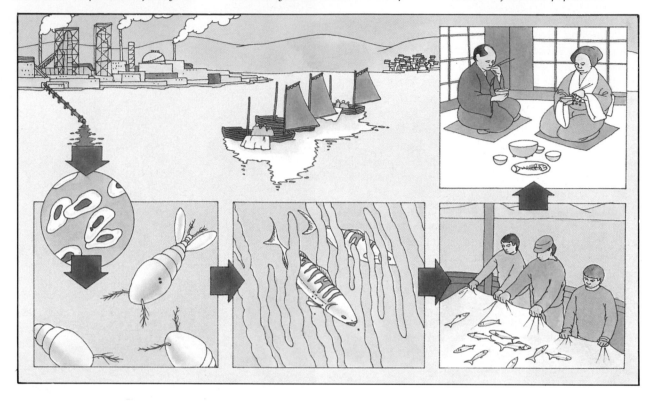

example in a permanently manned submarine base, would also be extremely wasteful in terms of energy and materials. Air tanks need refilling, and the alternative — air pumped from the surface — would be expensive in energy. A more elegant way of providing oxygen is being considered.

Taking nature as their model, materials technologists have devised a silicon-rubber substance that mimics the gills of a fish by "extracting" oxygen from water and exchanging it for carbon dioxide. The material is permeable to gases but not to water. Imagine a person on one side of it, and water on the other. As the person breathes the air, its concentration of oxygen falls while that of carbon dioxide rises. This puts the gas concentrations in the air out of equilibrium with the same gases dissolved in the water. So oxygen diffuses across the membrane from water to air, while carbon dioxide does the opposite. The result is a breathable atmosphere sustained at no cost, because fresh oxygen dissolves naturally from the water surface into the water itself and then into the breathed air.

Sustainable, self-powered solutions such as this are the only long-term answers to the problems of putting the human body where it was not designed to go. Theoretical plans for permanent space stations incorporate sealed ecosystems within. Water, nutrients, oxygen and carbon dioxide must all be recycled through the agency of crops, livestock and human inhabitants. Once set up, no extra raw materials would be needed. But there would be a need for an energy source to power the entire system. The heat and light from a nearby star would do nicely. And if this situation sounds familiar, it is because we are here already traveling through the galaxy on Spaceship Earth.

Trapped in the Web of Life

Human beings are an inevitable part of the web of life here on Earth. During the billions of years of our evolutionary past, animals and plants have adapted to the environment in order to survive. Humans are no exception to this rule. They have started a new trend, adapting the environment to themselves in order to prosper and apparently

One school of environmentalists argues that the increased use of fossil fuels will create a "greenhouse" effect — an increase in worldwide temperatures that would bring about the melting of the polar icecaps. The sea level would rise, with disastrous effects on the world's coastal cities. Opponents predict the opposite: a big freeze in which the world reverts to ice-age climatic conditions and the northern seas freeze over.

defying the laws of natural selection. It is an untried experiment and, as scientists are now learning, a hazardous route. This is so because of the interdependence of the natural systems with which they are tinkering. As they change one aspect of the environment to suit humans, its results will eventually tend to enlarge and have negative effects on other aspects. In many instances, this may ultimately feed back in the form of health threats.

One obvious example is atmospheric pollution. Over highly populated industrial cities, photochemical smog and smoke laden with soot and chemicals hang in the air, clogging people's lungs and worsening respiratory disorders such as bronchitis and emphysema. In the fall of 1948, seven thousand people in Donora, Pennsylvania became ill during a four-day fog, and the infamous London fog of 1952 was thought to be responsible for at least four thousand deaths in the city. In addition to the direct ill effects of inhalation, smog also contains chemicals such as peroxyacetyl nitrate that harm plant life. As the plants under the pall suffer, the animals that depend on them for food and shelter suffer too. Gradually, the whole living system is put out of balance.

Acid fumes from industrial smokestacks are another airborne pollutant. Often containing sulfur oxides, they become dissolved in atmospheric moisture to produce acid rain. So far, acid rain has had virtually no detectable direct effects on human health. But it does damage plant life wherever it falls. Entire forests in Scandinavia, central Europe, north-eastern Canada and some regions of the United States are being affected by this silent scourge.

The problem of air pollution in developed countries has, to some extent, been tackled successfully. In cities such as Los Angeles and Tokyo, the dangers are now less acute because of changes in car exhaust emission regulations, which severely limit the amounts of carbon monoxide and nitrogen and sulfur oxides in the exhaust. The gases are the chief pollutants in smog. The suffocating "pea-souper" fogs of London earlier this century have disappeared, thanks to the effectiveness of clean air legislation.

People are slow to learn from each others' ex-

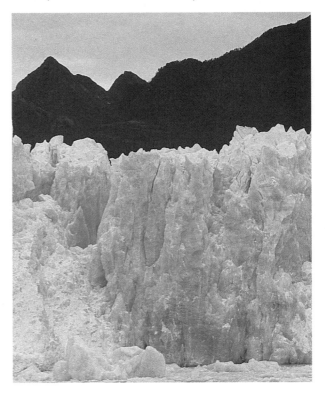

periences. What the first world did yesterday the second world does today, and the third world may well do tomorrow. Many cities in developing countries are beginning to suffer smogs from uncontrolled automobile emissions and permanent smoke clouds from the burning of charcoal and wood fires.

Another threat to health exists in the pollution of the environment by heavy metal elements. Lead, mercury, chromium, nickel and cadmium are clearly implicated as cancer-causing, and are thought to affect mental development in children. As chemically free, active forms in the environment they are a hazard to everyone. The metals come from lead additives in gasolene, industrial wastes, herbicides, pesticides and discarded consumer goods such as dead batteries.

Recently, a new group of deadly pollutants has come to light: the PCBs (polychlorinated biphenyls). These totally synthetic substances, now classed as carcinogens, are ingredients in many types of plastics, electrical equipment and engineering fluids. They hardly degrade naturally

According to many experts, the growth technology of the late twentieth century might not be computing, but bioengineering. In this Swiss laboratory, a prototype anticancer drug, created by manipulating the molecular arrangement of a particular protein, is being produced in a sterile environment. Stringent physical and chemical analysis will take place before animal trials are begun.

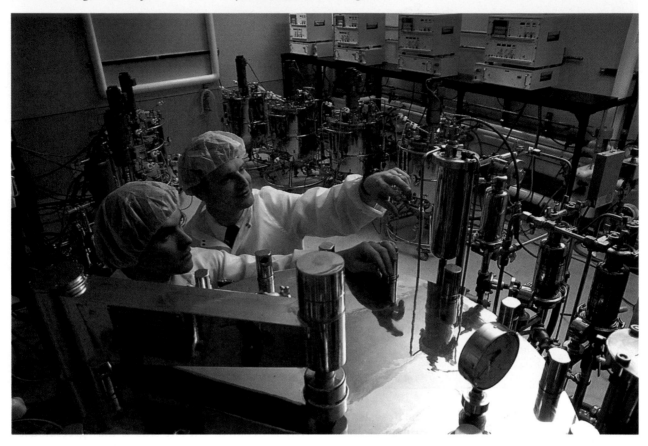

with potentially catastrophic implications as the polar icecaps begin to melt and major coastal cities around the world are gradually flooded.

The ice-agers, however, take the opposite view. Earth, they say, has always passed through cycles of warmth and cold, as evidenced by geological and fossil remains. Burning fossil fuels is only a minor variation in a major, unalterable fluctuation. The world is just leaving a "mini ice-age" that saw rivers such as the Thames in London freeze over regularly two or three centuries ago. But the long-term climatic trend is downward in terms of global temperatures, as the next ice age approaches.

Although much damage has already been done, there are some encouraging signs. Governments of industrialized nations are at last waking up to the harm and destruction, and plans are being formu-lated to get the ecosphere back into balance. These plans will doubtless gather momentum as their populations become directly affected.

One early and encouraging sign concerns the erosion of the ozone layer by chemicals such as fluorocarbons. Research using high-flying aircraft, high-altitude meteorological balloons and space vehicles has confirmed that some damage has already taken place. The United States is leading a movement to ban the culprit chemicals, before significant harm is done.

Science and technology could be used to solve many other problems that their ignorant use has created. One such area is the prediction of weather patterns, both locally and globally.

A Change in the Weather

Although human activities seem to be affecting the world's climatic stability, it may be feasible to make amends. One possibility would be to ma-nipulate the weather directly. At present scientists can do this only with uncertainty, on a very localized scale — and at huge cost. "Seeding"

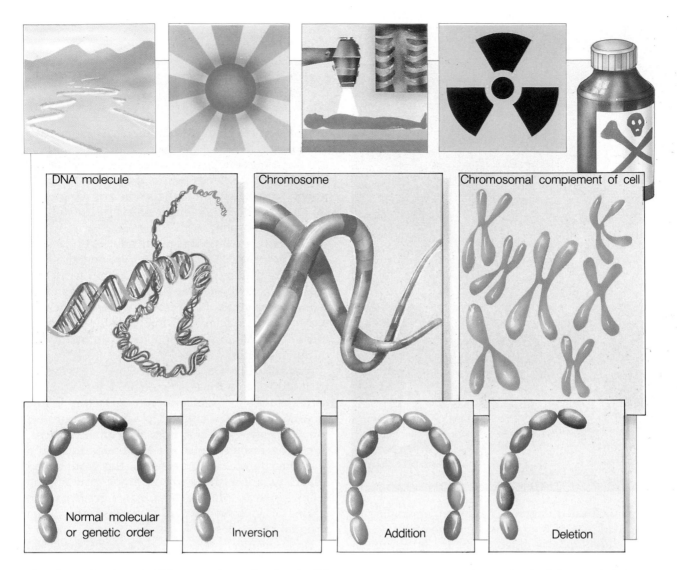

DNA molecule

Chromosome

Chromosomal complement of cell

Normal molecular or genetic order

Inversion

Addition

Deletion

clouds with silver iodide crystals or dry ice (solid carbon dioxide) probably increases rainfall; certain types of fog and hail can be minimized with a similar technique. But perhaps meteorologists cannot yet locate the critical "pressure points" for overall climatic change.

Currently meteorologists can forecast the weather with fair accuracy only four or five days in advance. Nevertheless, this allows them to give warnings and enable preparations to be put in place for hurricanes, monsoons, snow and other disruptive conditions, so saving human lives and property. Longer-term predictions will surely extend the accuracy as computer models of climatology advance.

Weather prediction is a fast-developing area. Remote-sensing satellites gather masses of data on layer temperatures, cloud cover and air movements. These are analyzed, by computer, together with data on terrestrial features, and to increasing-

Plant and animal characteristics are determined by the genetic content of their cells. A gene is the length of the chemical DNA (deoxyribonucleic acid) that encodes the production of a single protein. In organisms as complex as human beings there are thousands of such genes, linked together in chromosomes. If the order of the DNA in a gene is incorrect, or if the order of genes within a chromosome changes, mutations occur. This can happen naturally, possibly as the result of background radiation or the action of sunlight, or may be the result of exposure to artificial radiation, X rays, or certain chemicals.

115

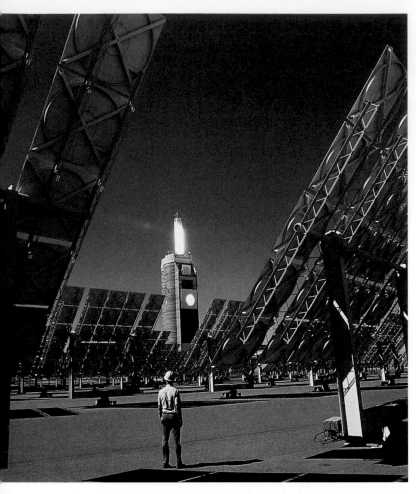

Theoretically, solar power is free and unlimited. But this unit, based in California, uses expensive high-tech computers. For poorer countries, cheaper, more applicable technologies may be preferable.

ly sophisticated degrees. As an understanding of the workings of the atmosphere increases, so critical situations may emerge where a little artificial input at a "pressure point" can create enormous change. This is analogous to selecting one finely-balanced boulder which is then tipped down a hill, where it generates an avalanche. Accurate modeling should be able to tell a scientist how big the avalanche will be and what course it will take, to obtain the desired effect.

Hurricanes, for instance, can now be identified at an early stage in their development. Computer modeling may one day be able to predict whether any specific embryo hurricane is going to pose a threat to humanity. Then, while it is still very "young," the hurricane could be diverted or forestalled by judicious use of non-polluting low-altitude explosives, detonated near its center. This technique would literally blow the hurricane off course, away from areas of population.

Tailoring the Body to the Environment

Bioscience may one day be able to help in the maintenance of future health by adapting the human body to changed conditions. There are two approaches. First are the "clip-on extras," such as gas filtration devices for inhaled air. These are not in the realm of science fiction; they are being used now by city cyclists and others who are at high risk of, and aware of, the danger posed by breathing a polluted atmosphere.

However, such an approach offers only a temporary solution. More permanently, geneticists of the future may be able to take nature in hand and alter the genetic makeup of human beings. This would raise difficult moral issues; nevertheless, techniques being developed now could have scientific end points in direct application to modifying our own species.

Agriculturists are already looking at ways to treat crop plants by genetic engineering, so as to increase their resistance to certain factors in the environment. For example, to adequately protect the Southern corn belt from pest plant species, American farmers must use herbicides in such a way that they tend to persist in the ground and adversely affect the soybean crops planted the following year. This has stimulated research into strains of soybean that are more resistant to the residual herbicides.

Until recently, workers could capitalize only on genes for herbicide resistance that are thrown up naturally by mutation — and thrown up in plants which can be hybridized with soybean (that is, are sexually compatible). Gene transfer technology should allow resistant genes to be isolated from a more distantly related plant species and "stitched" into the soybean's genes, so conferring on the soybean extra herbicide tolerance.

Genetic engineering has already progressed to the stage at which scientists can create highly modified new life forms in the laboratory. This short-circuits the natural mutation process on which evolution has relied in the past, and could provide tailor-made mutations. But it could also be hazardous. Previously most organisms evolved in harmony, or at least in some sort of balance, with each other. The sudden introduction of radically new organisms, without the lead time for other animals and plants to become acclimatized, could be catastrophic. It could also lead to the sudden extinction of species unable to compete with their new neighbors. Thorough ecological modeling would be needed for deciphering the consequences of such new introductions.

Genetic transfer may ultimately become applicable to humans. The appropriate genes for resistance to polluting chemicals, to low concentrations of oxygen in the atmosphere, or to high concentrations of carbon dioxide, would be identified in other animals. The genes would then be transferred to humans, presumably to the germ cells (egg and sperm) or at a very early stage of embryonic development. The moral and ethical issues of application will become significant topics of public discussion as the use of such techniques becomes more and more feasible.

In the shorter term, what of the next decade or two? There are many pressing problems to solve in the way humans relate to their environment. One of the basic aspects of this relationship is that the human body must consume an adequate, balanced diet in order to stay healthy. This diet should contain fats and carbohydrates for energy, proteins for tissue-building, and vitamins and minerals to maintain and regulate body functions. But for half a billion undernourished people in the world, this is at present an impossibility.

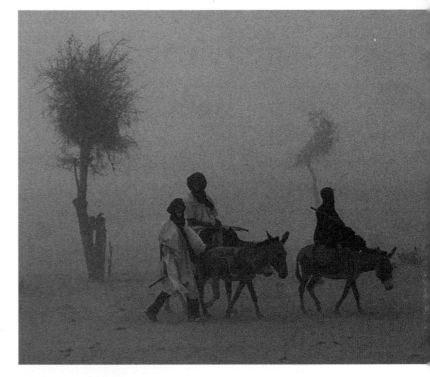

The Famine War

Theoretically, humankind possess the means to adequately feed every one of the four and a half billion people on earth; yet one human in nine goes hungry. A single Jumbo jet crash draws horror, grief and demands for extra safety. Yet malnutrition and its attendant diseases kill the equivalent of one Jumbo-load of passengers — nearly five hundred — every five minutes.

Food production in Africa has fallen overall by thirty per cent per person between 1970 and the early 1980s. One problem is post-harvest losses, which can run at fifty per cent and go as high as eighty per cent. Partly to blame are the modern high-yield crops. These harvest and keep well in the industrialized world, which has good grain storage facilities. But in Africa there are few such facilities and the new varieties, although high yielding even on minimal added artificial fertilizers, are nowhere nearly as resistant to post-harvest pests as are the local strains. The answer

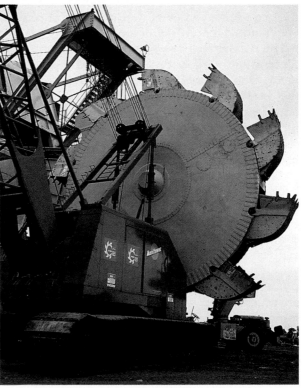

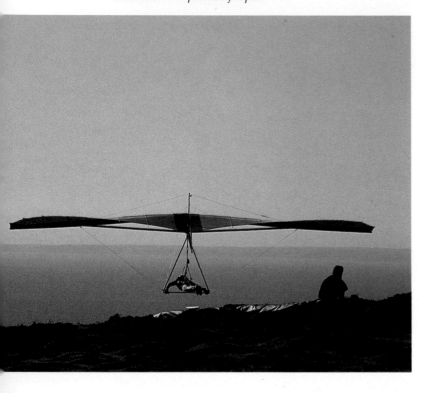

may be to develop even newer strains of cereals, better suited to local conditions.

The regions that can grow staple food crops are diminishing, largely because of land mismanagement. One of the biggest factors is desertification, the creation of arid areas by human activity. (It is not to be confused with desertization, the natural formation of arid regions.) More than thirty per cent of the world's land area, excluding the uninhabitable areas of the far north and south, is already desert, semi-desert, or on the way to becoming so. Five million acres of previously useful land, particularly in northern Africa and southern Asia, are lost each year. The chief causes of this continuing disaster are deforestation, over-cultivation and over-grazing, and poor irrigation. With sufficient will and resources, all of these processes could be reversed. Reafforestation programs, coupled if necessary with irrigation schemes, can make deserts fertile again.

To get to the bottom line, many people believe that the world's governments must act to put the global larder in order. Only when there is appropriate use of resources to grow and distribute food adequately can all humankind begin to move toward a brighter and healthier future.

The Personal Perspective

For inhabitants in the industrialized world, the major threats to health come mainly from modern eating habits and life styles. The very hallmarks of progress cause disease and death. The office worker drives to his or her office, sits at a desk all day, consumes high-fat, processed fast food, and encounters high-stress mental events with little opportunity for physical activity to work off the physiological effects of such a life style. The human body is certainly not designed for such an existence. Fortunately, since the 1970s, medical research has highlighted the major problems and offered solutions.

Few people in the developed countries remain unaware of such threats to their bodies. They include smoking tobacco, eating too much, eating too much saturated fatty acids (in animal products), eating too little fiber, being physically inactive, and not avoiding stress. These factors have been clearly demonstrated to damage health by many medical studies worldwide. One study of voluntary life-style changes in an entire community, Karelia in Finland (the "Flora Project"), has shown what is attainable: basically, less disease and more happiness.

Encouragingly, the thrust for increasingly healthy life styles is coming largely from the people. Most no longer want to be led by the hand; they demand both a say and a personal responsibility in their own health. Evidence is provided by the huge proliferation in sports participation, keep-fit clubs, gyms and the like. Joggers are a familiar sight in most neighborhoods. There is an increasing demand for food suppliers to provide more natural, unprocessed ingredients, because artificial additives, colorings and preservatives have been linked with such disorders as hyperactivity syndrome in children, headaches, and certain types of cancers. Health-food shops have opened in most towns, selling "natural" foods produced without the use of pesticides and herbicides, and processed without the addition of flavorings and other chemicals. Smoking, which along with obesity is one of the biggest contributors to ill health in modern

Alvin Toffler

Foretelling the Future

So much has happened to the world in the last eighty years or so — in terms of progress in technology, general science and the advance of knowledge — that some people have inevitably been left behind. Not only are they unable to fully comprehend the changes but they are incapable of coping with the rate at which those changes are being made. For those people, the condition they suffer from has been termed Future Shock — an expression that formed the title of a best-selling sociological critique, which remained seventy-eight weeks at the top of the US best-seller list, and was translated into more than nineteen languages. Its author was the journalist Alvin Toffler.

Toffler was born the son of a furrier in New York City in October 1928. Despite the wishes of his father that he should take up a legal career, journalism was his ambition from an early age. During his years at New York University, where he majored in English, Toffler set up and edited *Compass*, a literary periodical. After graduating in 1949 he was obliged, however, to take up various posts as an industrial laborer. This stood him in good stead when, in the early 1950s, he became editor of a small industrial journal, from which he moved on to join the staff of

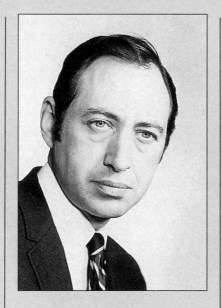

a newspaper.

By 1957 Toffler was in Washington D.C., working both freelance and for a small Pennsylvania daily as correspondent in the capital. At this point his speciality was political profiles. In 1960 he was employed by the magazine *Fortune* as associate editor and labor columnist — and it was for this publication that he put together the information that was later to be published as his first highly influential book, *The Culture Customers*; it was issued in late 1964. Toffler then spent the next five years assembling the material for *Future Shock*, which was published in mid-1970. Acclaim followed, since when he has worked on further articles and books

associated with ideas of the future, particularly in relation to education and politics.

At the heart of *The Culture Customers* is an account of the sudden wide expansion of cultural appreciation experienced by the general public, formerly the preserve only of the highbrow. Also central to the work is the reflection that such appreciation is still expanding even though official support — particularly financial — for artists and performers is diminishing equally rapidly.

In *Future Shock* he described himself as having been "born in the middle of human history" in that "as much has happened in the world since I was born as happened before." The result was, he said, that whereas former generations had had little choice in what to make of their lives, the present generation was undergoing "a paralyzing surfeit" of choices.

His later works have suggested, among other things, that education today must inevitably be out of date even as students graduate — for the world has changed again during their period of learning. Toffler is in considerable demand as a lecturer and guest speaker and, in contrast to the pessimism of some of his critics, the essence of his words is always optimistic.

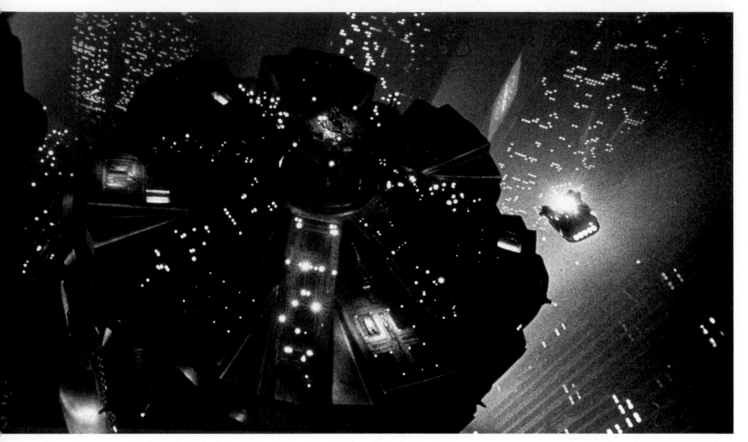

society, is at last declining in incidence in virtually every country in the Western world. Classes in relaxation and stress relief have never been fuller.

The results of this new awareness are showing themselves in the health statistics. For instance, the mortality rate from heart disease in the United States is now falling significantly. In middle-aged and elderly American males, the rate was 800 deaths per hundred-thousand in 1968; by 1985 it was approaching 500. Coronary mortality rates are also declining in Australia, Belgium, Finland, New Zealand, Norway, and elsewhere. In Britain the rate of cardiovascular disorders (and, significantly, of cigarette smoking) is still high: coronary heart disease kills one person every four minutes. But the early signs of improvement are there.

Health educators are acutely aware of one particular aspect of their work: how can they change the habits of all sectors of the population, across the socioeconomic spectrum? The decline of cigarette smoking in the United States happened first among the professional and semi-professional groups. Dietary improvements are following a similar pattern. Manual workers have proved more "resistant" to media information concerning general health hazards. There is concern among some that continuation of this difference in attitudes may deepen the rich-poor divide, driving an even larger wedge between the "healthy wealthy" and the "sickly poor."

To prevent this split, planners are identifying those groups in which resistance to health education is high. They then try to reach these segments of the population through their dominant entertainment/information medium — in most cases, broadcast television. Slots for health promotion "advertising" are booked into prime-time. Stars from sport and the soap operas are engaged to put over the message. In advertising jargon, the "C through D/Es are being targeted" — that is, the advantages of a healthy body and a healthy environment are being "sold" to socioeconomic classes C, D and E.

The media are also being used to warn young people about potential health hazards, particularly those than can result from alcohol or drug abuse. These approaches cost far more than old-fashioned techniques such as free leaflets distributed at the public library. But health educators hope the benefits will also show a corresponding increase.

A Dark Vision of the Future

The blockbusting movie *Bladerunner* painted a bleak picture of future society. Set on America's West Coast a few decades hence, dark raining skies lower above crumbling cities crammed with people. The wealthy and able have moved away from Earth altogether, to "off-world" colonies that are the planetary equivalents of today's privileged city garden suburbs. Enormous sky-borne billboards advertise the fairytale life that an off-worlder, living in an artificial environment designed to be perfect for humans, can expect. Meanwhile, the environment on Earth is slowly but nevertheless continually degenerating. Only the poor, disabled, unhealthy and those of lower intelligence remain. Pollution, overcrowding, hunger and disease are on the increase. There has been no solution to the resource shortage, no solution to the energy crisis.

Such a scenario is of little credit to a species that sets itself above others in the animal kingdom in terms of intelligence, understanding, compassion and ability to influence the future. The planet that bore *Homo sapiens* is humankind's only true home. As such, people ought to be ensuring that its environment is kept clean and self-sustaining and that a worldwide ecological balance is established and maintained for all living creatures. All humans will then be able to look forward to some sort of future health and happiness, to some sort of continuing harmony between themselves and their surroundings. In grappling with such colossal difficulties, science and technology — which have arguably helped create much of the problem — must form the basis of the solution. They must do so in concert with clearly delineated moral and political views.

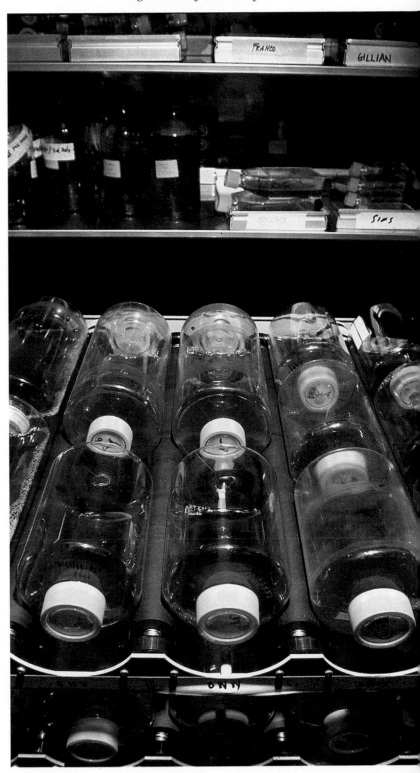

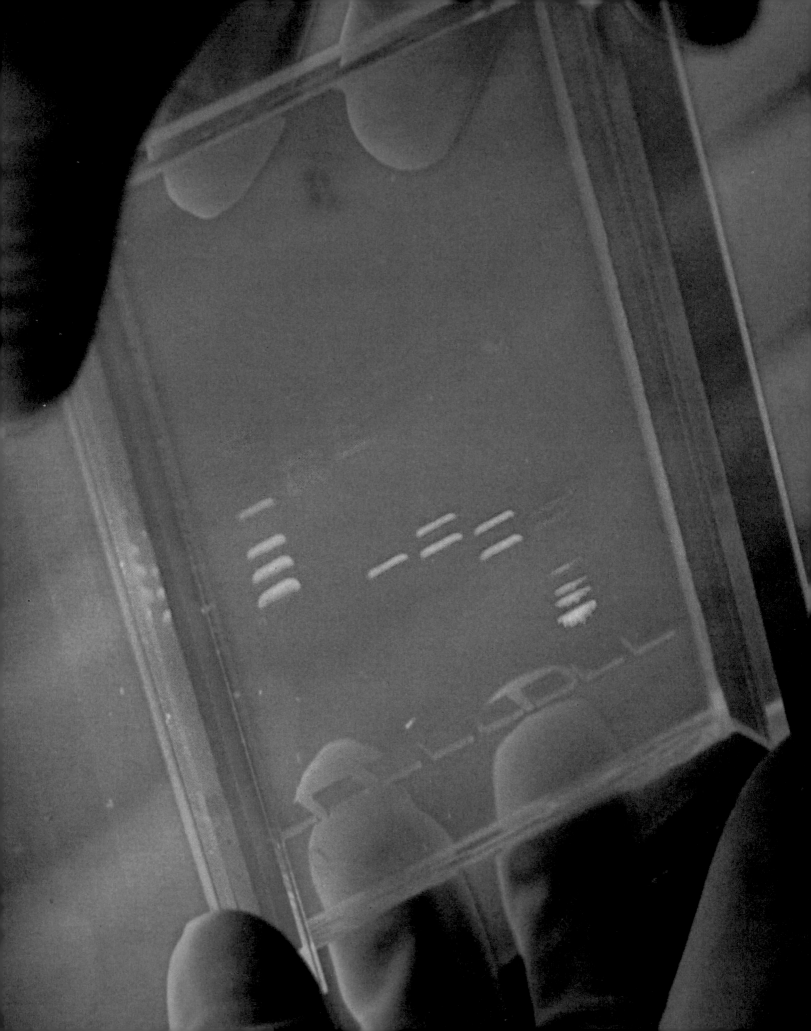

Chapter 6

Health in the Future

In the space of a single generation, many people in the United States have become firm believers in the value of exercise. "Fit for life" is just one of many phrases that have become popular in the 1980s. People aware of the new trend in fitness can be seen running along beaches or around city blocks, swimming, stretching and exerting themselves to achieve greater suppleness in their bodies. Yet despite the apparent national belief in the benefits of exercise, a study from the Federal Government in 1985 showed that most young or middle-aged people still confine themselves to nothing more strenuous than pushing a shopping trolley around a supermarket or pushing buttons to change channels on the television. In other words, most Americans are not as fit as they think they are.

A survey by the Office of Disease Prevention and Health Promotion at the US Department of Health and Human Services (HHS) showed that between eighty and ninety per cent of Americans do not exercise enough to benefit their health. Sufficient exercise is defined as an activity that boosts heart and lung performance to sixty per cent or more of its capacity at least three times a week for a full twenty minutes; this is the minimum needed to produce significant cardiovascular benefit. In 1980 the Public Health Service urged that by 1990, one-half of the over-sixty-fives and three-fifths of the under-sixty-fives should be achieving such a standard. However, the 1985 figures suggest that the likelihood is small that such a goal might be reached.

In addition to the national lack of exercise, just under one-third of men and more than one-third of women are heavier than the recommended weight for their age, height and build. And there has been no significant change in the statistics since the mid-1970s. Even though it became known that regular exercise could improve the performance of the heart and consequently reduce the risk of heart disease — with the result that

Resembling lights on an electronic control panel, genes from bacteria undergo gel electrophoresis. This process, which enables the separation of fragments of DNA, prepares the genes for insertion into mammalian cells. In this way, the cells can be custom engineered for the creation of potential new pharmaceutical products, including tailor-made drugs and vaccines.

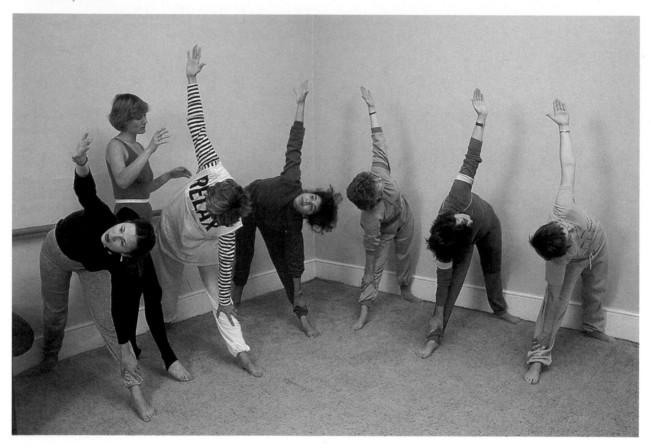

billions of dollars have been spent on fitness —
the proportion of people who are active has
remained the same.

When people find themselves victims of poor
health, whether through acute, chronic, degenerative or genetic disorders, they tend to expect the
medical profession to help them out. As epidemi-
ological studies provide more evidence for the
possible environmental and dietary cause of illness, the medical profession will be increasingly
relied upon to provide a passport to continued
health. One area that could certainly benefit from
development of appropriate technology to maintain health is heart disease—still the largest
single cause of death in the United States.

Heartening News

The incredible efficiency of the human heart is
something that is easy to take for granted. This
small organ — about the size of a man's fist —
continuously pumps large quantities of blood
around the circulatory system with no rest periods
longer than a fraction of a second. A healthy heart
moves ten tons of blood each day for a lifetime. It
is supremely efficient, adjusting energy consumption and pumping rate from about six watts when
the body is at rest to twenty-five watts or so when
fully active. In a resting person, the heartbeat
accounts for around twenty-five per cent of the
body's energy consumption. But the failure of this
one critical organ leads to death. Science is rapidly
advancing to offer hope to those with failing hearts
in two ways. These are heart transplantation,
using a natural heart donated by someone who has
just died, and the development of the completely
artificial heart.

The first artificial heart to be implanted in a
human was built by the American scientist Dr.
Robert Jarvik. In 1982, surgeon William de Vries
implanted it into a 62-year-old Seattle dentist,

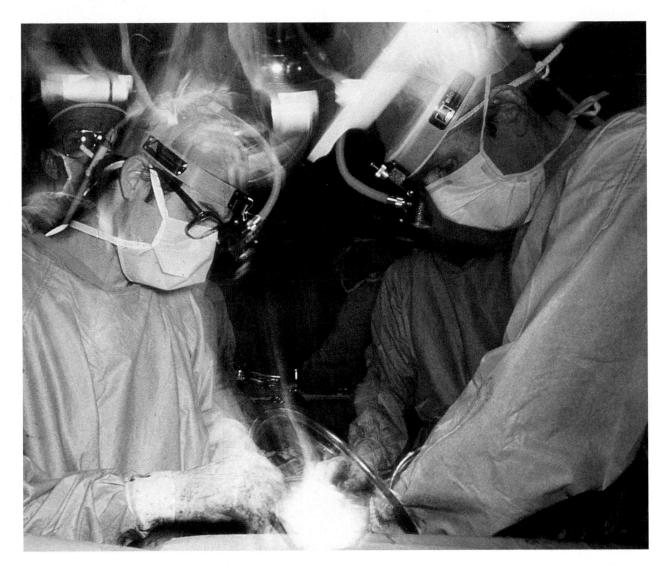

Barney Clark, who then lived on for another 112 days. (Death was caused by the failure of other organs damaged before the operation.)

Further implants of mechanical hearts have shown that patients can adapt to them. However, it will be some time before it is known how the life expectancy of people fitted with such artificial devices is increased, and how the quality of life can be improved.

One of the problems with the Jarvik heart (known as the Jarvik 7) is the incidence of clotting in the patient's blood system soon after the transplant. Blood that sticks to the inside surfaces of the artificial heart tends to be washed off in small lumps or clots. Despite the administration of clot-preventing drugs to patients, some clots do not dissolve before reaching the brain. There they may lodge in small blood vessels, blocking the flow of blood and starving parts of the brain of oxygen. The tragic result is a stroke.

The recipient of an artificial heart is linked by tubes to the apparatus that will power his new organ. The tubes carry "pulses" of compressed air, which bring about the pumping action of the heart. Scientists are now working on a self-contained artificial heart driven by atomic power, which will allow the recipient total freedom of movement.

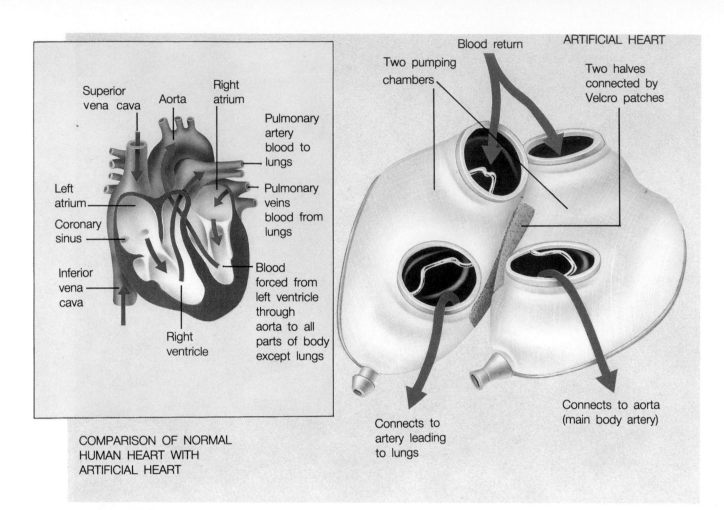

Blood return

Two pumping chambers

Two halves connected by Velcro patches

Connects to aorta (main body artery)

Connects to artery leading to lungs

Superior vena cava

Aorta

Right atrium

Pulmonary artery blood to lungs

Pulmonary veins blood from lungs

Left atrium

Coronary sinus

Blood forced from left ventricle through aorta to all parts of body except lungs

Inferior vena cava

Right ventricle

COMPARISON OF NORMAL HUMAN HEART WITH ARTIFICIAL HEART

On December 2, 1982, Barney Clark was the first human recipient of the Jarvik artificial heart. Its size, weight and function — with one side of two similarly constructed halves pumping blood to the lungs, and the other to the rest of the body — are equivalent to those of a natural heart. The pumping action of a normal heart occurs as a result of the inherent rhythmic contractions of the cardiac muscle. In the artificial heart (right), the pumping action is achieved by compressed air pressing against a rubber diaphragm and forcing the blood through the valve into the circulation (far right). This is dependent on an external drive system timing device weighing 375 pounds, connected to the artificial heart by two six-foot tubes that leave the recipient's chest.

The Pennsylvania State Heart, developed by the surgeon Dr. William Pierce, was designed to take into account the Jarvik problems. It is made with smooth and seamless chambers for blood, and valves entirely of plastic. These modifications reduce the chance of blood sticking to the walls of the heart and of subsequent clotting. Unlike the Jarvik 7, the Pennsylvania State Heart heart has an automatic blood-flow regulator, which allows it to compensate for any extra pumping the body needs during exertion.

There remain, however, a number of difficulties associated with the artificial heart. One is that the mechanical heart, which is around the same weight but slightly bigger than a normal heart, has to be powered by compressed air. This is ducted by unwieldy tubes from a large bedside machine through a hole in the patient's chest. Smaller portable power units are being developed, which will be carried like a shoulder bag. Such units are vital if people with artificial hearts are to enjoy anything like a normal life.

At present, long-term survival with an artificial heart is unlikely — although Dr. Jarvik believes

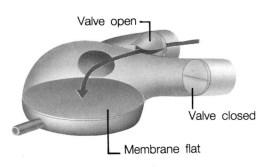

Valve open
Valve closed
Membrane flat

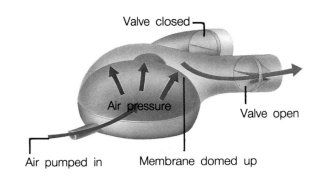

Valve closed
Air pressure
Valve open
Air pumped in
Membrane domed up

some 25,000 people will have them by the mid-1990s. Where mechanical hearts should be able to score a significant success is in conjunction with heart transplant programs. Heart transplants are becoming increasingly common as better drugs are introduced to combat the tissue rejection problems that dogged early operations of this type. Around seventy per cent of patients now survive the first year with a remarkably improved quality of life, and for those surviving for more than one year the chance of living more than five years is about ninety per cent. New and even better drugs should help to increase these figures. But the drawback with transplantation is the time it takes for a suitable donor organ to become available. One way to overcome the problem is to use the mechanical heart as a stopgap, to keep the patient alive until a natural donor heart for transplantation becomes available.

In September 1985, twenty-five-year-old Michael Drummond was the first to benefit in this way. A viral disease had attacked his heart and he would have died but for the implantation of a Jarvik heart. Nine days later a natural heart became available and was successfully transplanted. The mechanical heart could also lead, in time, to a great advance in avoiding the problems of rejection associated with less than ideal, hurried tissue matches with some transplanted hearts.

Beating Diabetes

Another sort of disability is typified by diabetes mellitus. In this disease, failure of the pancreas to produce insulin leads to loss of control over body glucose levels. The discovery of a method of introducing insulin so that patients no longer need to inject themselves daily would be highly desirable. Some diabetics have already been given an insulin pump, which comprises a small electric pump linked to a tube under the skin that injects insulin into the bloodstream.

Improved technology has reduced the size of these external infusion pumps, but what diabetics would most like is freedom from the commitment to daily doses of insulin. The fulfilment of this dream rests with a small glucose sensor currently being developed. If such a sensor could accurately monitor blood glucose levels, which change throughout the day depending on the amount of physical exertion, and on what and how much a person eats, and relay this information to an insulin-releasing mechanism, then a complete device could be inserted beneath the diabetic's skin. Simply topping up the insulin would be the only regular commitment needed by the patient. Another advantage would be that the diabetic could achieve much better glucose control, with insulin being released into the bloodstream only as and when the body needed it.

Immunity to Multiple Sclerosis

Another disabling condition is multiple sclerosis (MS), a chronic disease of the nervous system in which areas of hardened and defective tissue appear at random in the brain and spinal cord. But hope for a future cure comes from scientists at Stanford University, California, whose work on mice is extremely encouraging for future treatment of the condition in humans.

In laboratory animals injected with spinal cord material from other mice, a reaction occurs against both the foreign material and against their own

Providing a potential source of relief for diabetes sufferers, the insulin pump maintains a virtually normal level of blood sugar (green line), without recourse to daily injections of insulin. The pump detects the blood

sugar level by means of a special needle inserted into a vein. When blood sugar is low, as it is before eating (A), little or no insulin is released by the pump. After eating (B) there is a dramatic increase in the

level of blood sugar, and insulin is released accordingly. For the two hours following eating (C to E), blood sugar level gradually decreases and insulin release is made to fall off almost completely.

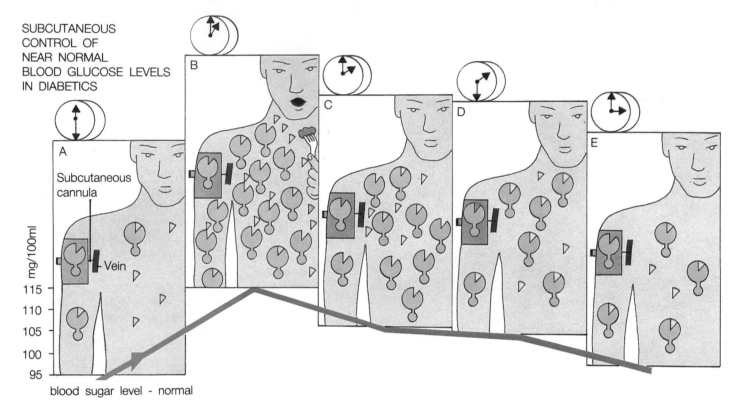

SUBCUTANEOUS CONTROL OF NEAR NORMAL BLOOD GLUCOSE LEVELS IN DIABETICS

Subcutaneous cannula

Vein

mg/100ml

115
110
105
100
95

blood sugar level - normal

spinal cord. This is an autoimmune reaction, a reaction against the body which the immune system is supposed to be defending. Multiple sclerosis is believed also to be an autoimmune disease in which, for some reason, the patient's immune system turns against the brain and nervous system. The condition induced in mice — known as experimental allergic encephalomyelitis (EAE) — is thus a model for MS.

The Stanford team have managed to develop a treatment that stops the onset of EAE symptoms and reverses them in mice in which they have already developed. The team identified a class of blood cells responsible for the EAE reaction in mice. The cells are a subclass of the type of white cell called T-cells, whose normal function is to strengthen immune reactions against foreign agents entering the body. The cells were rendered inactive by promoting the formation of antibodies against them, and the mice were cured. The Stanford researchers reported that "the successful treatment of mouse EAE suggests that therapy

with monoclonal antibodies to the human equivalent might prove effective in the treatment of MS and perhaps other diseases in which T-cell subsets play a role." It may be some years before they know if they are right. Meanwhile, MS sufferers are provided with some hope.

Detecting Genetic Defects

A whole range of conditions disabling to the body or mind are the result of genetic defects present from birth. Most genetic disorders are incurable; many are progressive and fatal. Such defects can be detected in fetuses during pregnancy by such techniques as chorionic villus sampling and amniocentesis. The first involves taking a sample of cells from the chorion, one of the membranes surrounding the fetus. In amniocentesis, the amniotic fluid in which the fetus "floats" is sampled. If an abnormality is detected, the option of an abortion can be offered to the parents, and in this way the prevalence of the more serious defects may be steadily reduced. New techniques are enabling more and more such defects to be detected before birth.

A British team at Oxford University announced in the fall of 1985 that they had developed the first-ever test to identify polycystic kidney disease, a serious defect that eventually demands the need for renal dialysis (treatment using a kidney machine). The team discovered the precise gene defect responsible for the condition and identified a so-called "marker" for that defect.

A marker is a length of DNA — the primary genetic material — with specific features known to be characteristic of people with a particular genetic defect, and never (or very seldom) found in people without the defect. When such a known marker is found during an analysis of cellular material, doctors know that there is a high probability that the person or fetus concerned carries the genetic defect, even before there is outward evidence of the results of faulty gene action.

The researchers at Oxford actually found two markers for polycystic kidney disease, which gives them a ninety-five per cent chance of spotting a potential victim.

In the future this will allow parents-to-be to know when they face a ninety-five per cent chance of giving birth to an affected fetus.

Similarly, an American team has moved closer to pinpointing the precise genetic defect responsible for the serious and crippling disease Duchenne muscular dystrophy (DMD), which involves weakness and a gradual wasting away of muscles. Some markers for the condition are already known, but they are not very reliable. Researchers at the Children's Hospital, Boston, have managed to considerably narrow down the general area on the chromosome in which the defective gene is known to be located. They have done this by finding a new marker nearer the target gene than the marker used previously. The location of this marker should also make the genetic test for DMD more reliable. By the end of the 1980s, the actual defective gene will probably be precisely pinpointed. Thus the two-thirds of all cases of DMD defects that are hereditary can theoretically be detected at an early stage, and prospective parents given the option of abortion.

Once the defective gene responsible for a condi-

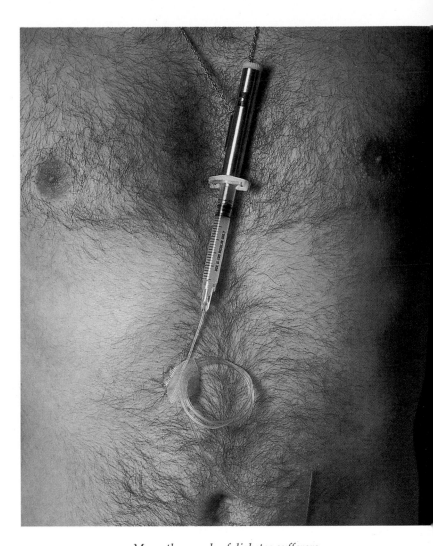

Many thousands of diabetes sufferers wear miniature pumps which can deliver a steady stream of insulin through a narrow tube inserted into a vein. This method produces fewer long-term diabetic complications than when insulin is given by comparatively large daily injections.

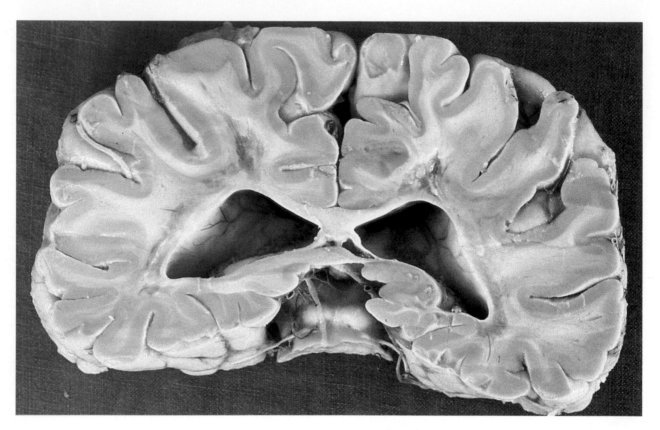

Affected by multiple sclerosis, this scarred brain has been a victim of the body's own immune system. Experiments with antibodies that reverse such autoimmune reactions may prove effective in the treatment and prevention of this debilitating disorder.

tion has been identified, it is now possible to take a sample of DNA from a fetus using the chorionic villus sampling technique. The sample can be matched with another piece of DNA from a "library" to see if it carries the fault. If it does, then an abortion can be offered.

The Gene Machine and Its Engineers

To many people abortion is not, however, a satisfactory option. Gene therapy is now on the horizon as an alternative, and may eventually enable people to be "cured" of the effects of their defective gene or genes. Genetic engineers at a number of American laboratories are currently preparing to embark on the first trials of human gene therapy. This promises to be a revolutionary approach to the treatment of inherited disorders such as Lesch-Nyhan syndrome, a condition caused by a single gene defect which manifests itself as paralysis and mental retardation.

The plan of such trials is to inject healthy, normal copies of the gene into the bone marrow

Medical science has taken giant strides toward isolating the gene that causes cystic fibrosis — a hereditary disorder that is fatal in children and young adults. With cloning techniques made possible by genetic engineering, researchers use probes — short pieces of human DNA — to seek out the gene for the disorder. They hope also to develop tests for diagnosing cystic fibrosis before birth and for detecting carriers.

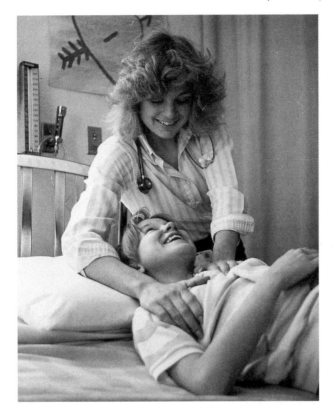

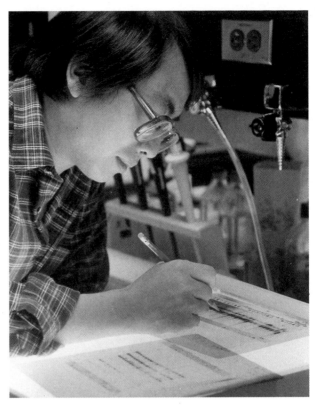

cells of a victim of a genetic disorder. In Lesch-Nyhan syndrome the gene defect prevents cells from producing the enzyme hypoxanthine-guanine phosphoribosyl transferase (HPRT), which is needed to metabolize basic compounds. It is hoped that the implanted "good" genes will begin producing large enough quantities of the enzyme to cure the disease.

One problem facing scientists carrying out the first steps in the new genetic revolution is how to design an efficient delivery system, or vector, for getting the gene into cells. Ideally scientists would like to target the stem cells. These are immature bone marrow cells that divide and develop into red and white blood cells. They also include many of the "housekeeping" cells so important in producing vital enzymes. But stem cells are the rarest and most elusive in the bone marrow. The next best result researchers hope to achieve is to get the foreign genes into all the cells in a marrow sample, and thereby possibly hit a few stem cells.

To achieve this marriage of cellular materials, scientists have been using one of nature's most successful invaders, the virus. For example, one technique being developed makes use of a mouse leukemia virus. The gene that controls the virus's replication process is chemically removed by the scientists and replaced with an equivalent human gene, together with appropriate signals for its regulation.

Several million marrow cells are extracted from mouse bones and incubated with the viral vector, which deposits its genes in the nucleus of every marrow cell within forty-eight hours. A mouse is then subjected to irradiation to destroy its resident marrow cells, leaving space for new marrow growth. The altered marrow cells are injected into the marrow space, and the as yet unspecialized stem cells start to grow and to repopulate the bone. Several research groups believe they are close to getting the inserted genes expressed in such experimental mice.

Once there is proof that such gene therapy works efficiently, it may become available for the

A revolutionary approach to conquering inherited disorders, particularly those involving faulty enzyme production, involves injecting healthy copies of the relevant gene into the bone marrow of an affected person. The "good" genes should then begin to produce enough of the missing enzyme to cure the disease. If initial trials are successful, the method could provide hope for thousands of patients.

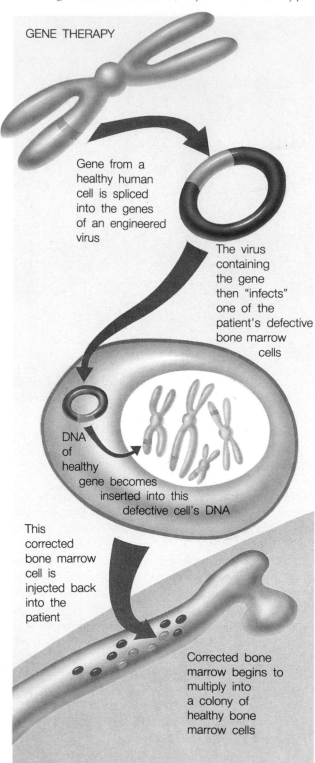

GENE THERAPY

Gene from a healthy human cell is spliced into the genes of an engineered virus

The virus containing the gene then "infects" one of the patient's defective bone marrow cells

DNA of healthy gene becomes inserted into this defective cell's DNA

This corrected bone marrow cell is injected back into the patient

Corrected bone marrow begins to multiply into a colony of healthy bone marrow cells

benefit of people suffering from severe genetic disorders. The first targets of such gene therapy will probably be three extremely rare diseases which affect only around ten births in a million. The diseases are Lesch-Nyhan syndrome, whose symptoms include physical and mental retardation; adenosine deaminase deficiency, an enzyme disorder of the type that killed the famous "bubble boy"; and purine nucleoside phosphorylase deficiency, another immune system disorder. In all three of these cases, the human genes responsible have been isolated and studied, which means that the relevant defective genes can, in theory, be replaced.

As researchers learn more about gene regulation, they may start tackling more complicated disorders such as cystic fibrosis, sickle-cell anemia, diabetes, and even cancer. The application of genetic engineering techniques to humans has authoritarian overtones to some people. But these misgivings are dismissed by the scientists concerned, who quickly point out that the new therapies are to be used only on body cells and will not alter the sex cells involved in reproduction and hence cannot affect future generations.

Genetic analysis also promises to yield a kind of genetic prophecy, identifying natural predispositions to some disorders. The list might include breast or colon cancer, diabetes, depression, schizophrenia and a form of early senility known as Alzheimer's disease. The greater scientists' knowledge of genetics becomes, so more genetic links to these conditions will be identified in the form of defective genes or groups of genes. The advantage of knowing at an early age whether a child is likely to be predisposed to a particular condition later in life is that a preventive life style can be adopted. For instance, geneticists predict that they will shortly be able to identify genes predisposing people to heart disease. Dietary and drug intervention could help people with such genes to put off or prevent heart disease.

Mastery Over Malaria

Genetic technology will probably be instrumental in the development of new and better vaccines against disease. For instance, more than one million people die of malaria each year in Africa alone,

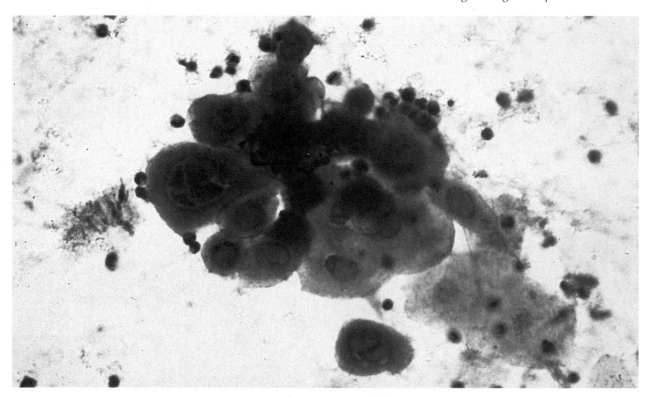

most of them children under five. Campaigns to reduce the incidence of malaria by controlling the mosquitoes that spread the disease, or through the use of drugs, have generally failed. Malaria is on the increase in several countries.

Malaria is caused by various species of *Plasmodium*, a single-celled organism that lives as a parasite in the red cells of the blood. It is contracted when a person is bitten by an Anopheles mosquito carrying the parasite, which it transmits through its saliva. Two to five weeks later, the victim has a sudden shivering attack and his or her temperature soars to at least 104°F. Vomiting and a headache often accompany the fever, which recur every two or three days.

Until recently, the major problem with making a life-saving vaccine against malaria was that the malarial parasites, which cause the disease, could not be grown outside the body on a large scale. Genetic engineers have now cloned antigens from the surface of the parasites, by isolating the genes for the antigens and transplanting them into bacteria. The bacteria are then grown into huge cultures and used to produce malarial parasite antigens on a large scale.

When the antigen material was injected into rabbits and mice it produced antibodies against the malaria antigen. This strongly suggests that a vaccine made in this way for humans would have a similar effect. One aim is to produce vaccines that contain several different antigens, corresponding to the several different developmental stages of the malarial parasite in the human body (all of which have different antigens). Such vaccines could be effective in wiping out all malaria's parasitic forms. As a result, public health workers would have a powerful tool for controlling this serious and debilitating disease.

Liberation from Leprosy

With malaria, leprosy is one of the scourges of Africa, affecting between ten and fifteen million people. There are two main forms of the disease. Tuberculoid leprosy involves the nerve endings, causing gradual loss of sensation, paralysis and pale areas on the skin. In lepromatous leprosy,

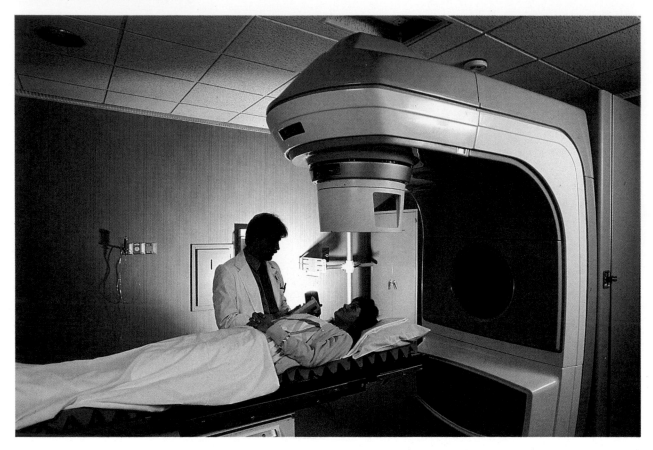

patches of skin lose their pigmentation and there may be ulceration of the membranes lining the nose, mouth and throat. Leprosy can usually be treated, but patients with the severe disabling form of the disease — lepromatous leprosy — may have to take the drug dapsone for the rest of their lives to avoid a relapse. Resistance to the drug is spreading, however, and there is therefore an urgent need to produce a vaccine. Before the mid-1980s it was impossible to make such a vaccine because there was no method of growing the leprosy bacillus.

Dr. Richard Young and his colleagues at Biomedical Research in Cambridge, Massachusetts, and researchers at other centers, have isolated specific genes that represent the genetic blueprints for a number of surface antigens of the leprosy bacillus. (Antigens are the protein substances that stimulate the body's defenses to produce antibodies.) These genes have been implanted into

viruses that infect and multiply in the common laboratory bacterium *Escherichia coli*, reproducing the antigens in the process. Five different leprosy bacillus antigens have been produced using this technique. The scientists hope that in the next few years they will discover the antigens that will stimulate immunity against the leprosy bacillus. This would enable the production of an effective vaccine that could be made in much larger quantities and much more cheaply than the present experimental vaccine (which is grown in armadillos—a laborious and expensive process).

A Vaccine Against Venereal Disease

A commercial vaccine may also soon be available against gonorrhea. It is a bacterial infection, caused by a gonococcus which usually enters the body along the urethra (the tube that carries urine out of the bladder). A week after contracting the disease, a man may notice a discharge of pus from

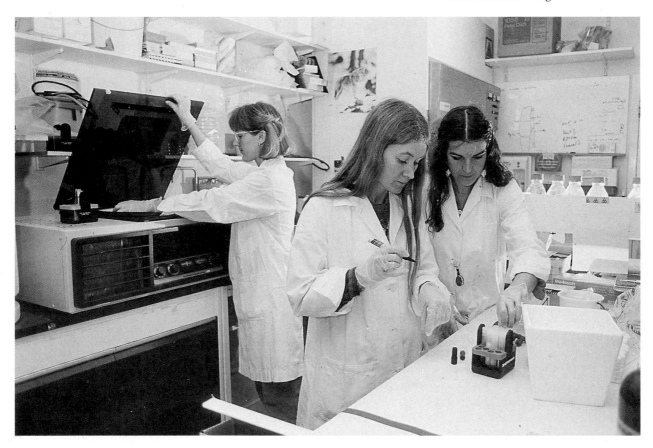

the penis and have a burning feeling during urination. Symptoms take about a week longer to appear in women, and may be so mild that they pass unnoticed.

This sexually-transmitted disease, widespread throughout the world, is reaching epidemic proportions in Africa and south-eastern Asia. In parts of western Africa, one-quarter of the women are infertile by the age of twenty-five as a result of gonorrhea infection. At present the only treatment is with antibiotics, to many of which resistance is developing.

Dr. Gary Schoolink and his colleagues at Stanford University have been trying to produce a gonorrhea vaccine. They have discovered a protein on the "coat" of the gonorrhea bacterium which, if isolated and brought into contact with an animal's cells, produces antibodies. Trials are underway to see if the isolation of this protein antigen will lead to the development of an effective vaccine. The vaccine should be relatively cheap to produce because the specific protein is comparatively simple and can be made by direct laboratory chemical synthesis. Scientists believe a commercial vaccine may be available by 1990.

Steps Against Cystitis

Protein isolation has also been instrumental in the development of a potential vaccine for cystitis, an unpleasant urinary tract inflammation which affects an estimated fifteen per cent of all women at some time in their lives. It causes frequent urination, which involves a painful burning sensation. Backache and fever are also common symptoms. Scientists at Stanford University have produced benign strains of a bacterium that causes cystitis, and engineered it to produce the protein which the cystitis strain uses to attack urinary tract cells. The protein can be produced in large quantities and is easy to purify. It has proved an effective

Robert K. Jarvik
Artificial Hearts

The present most successful form of surgery involving replacement of a human heart is that in which both the heart and the lungs of a recently brain-dead donor are transplanted into a needy recipient. But in the near future the frequency of this exceedingly complex and long operation is likely to decrease in favor of two other surgical methods. First is transplantation of a donor's heart alone, an operation not now common in the United States. Such transplantation is likely to become more assured of success as techniques combating tissue rejection and other complications rapidly improve.

Second, the perfecting of the artificial heart may be expected by the mid-1990s. Already various models have been used satisfactorily for periods of more than a year at a time. In each case, however, much of the machinery involved has had to remain external to the patient. Apparently unrelated additional symptoms have occurred in patients fitted with such a heart, some of them independently fatal. The artificial heart in its present form is thus most suited to emergency and temporary heart replacement. The next frontier is to invent a heart that does not lead to complications. And the person most likely to cross that

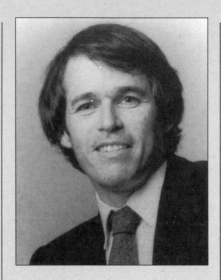

frontier is the brilliant inventor-physician Dr. Robert Jarvik.

Robert Koffler Jarvik was born the son of a physician in Midland, Michigan, in May 1946 shortly before the family moved to Stamford, Connecticut. Dexterous and inventive even as a teenager, his experience in assisting his father during surgery led him to devise improvements to some of the surgical equipment. On leaving school he attended Syracuse University, New York State. Initially he specialized in architecture, but he later switched to a medical course when it was discovered that his father was suffering from a heart condition. His degree, received in 1968, was in zoology. This meant that Jarvik had not, at this date, completed sufficient medical work to justify his acceptance at any US college for a doctorate course. So he spent two years at an Italian University school of medicine, and on his return was accepted by New York University — from which his master's degree came in 1971.

That same year saw him working under the direction of Dr. Willem Kolff — an equally inventive physician — at the University of Utah's Institute for Biomedical Engineering, where the first artificial heart was in the process of design.

He joined the heart project enthusiastically and creatively; experimentation following Jarvik's ideas led to rapid advances over the next six years. Then, in December 1982, a retired dentist named Barney Clark became the first recipient of "Jarvik 7", the first truly operational artificial heart, as a result of surgery lasting well over seven hours.

Other artificial heart transplantations followed. Most successful was that on William J. Schroeder, who received an improved "Jarvik 7" in November 1984 and lived on for twelve months in spite of a crippling stroke eighteen days after the operation.

A refined, fully portable artificial heart ("Jarvik 8") is likely to be brought into use during 1986 or 1987.

Victims of leprosy (below) sit weakened by the disease which attacks the nerves of the face, arms and legs. Most alarming are the disabling deformities that occur as the disease progresses, but which may be prevented if drugs are administered in the early stages. The use of drugs is, however, becoming less effective as patients grow resistant to them, and the search for an effective new vaccine is underway. By isolating the substance in the genes that stimulates immunity against leprosy, scientists hope to devise a vaccine that will be cheaper and easier to produce than that presently grown in armadillos (below right).

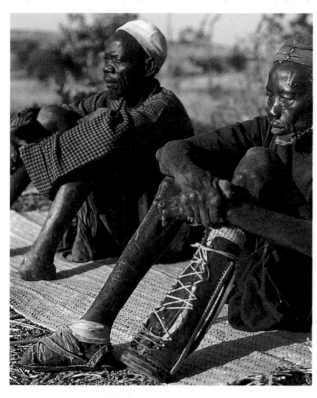

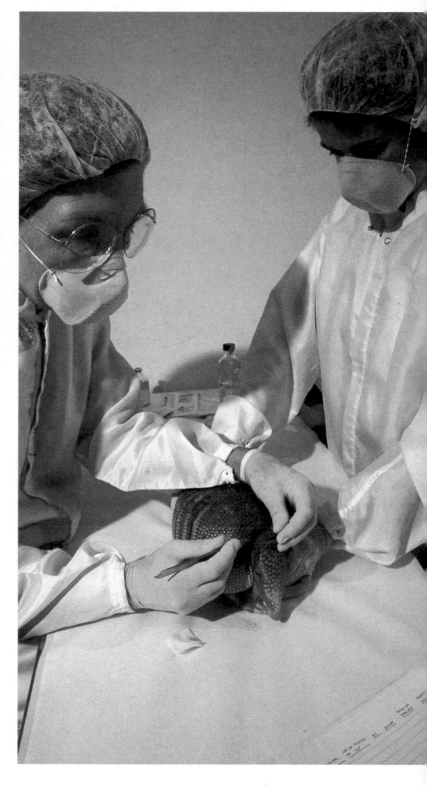

vaccine in mice, and a commercial vaccine for use on humans could be available by the end of the 1980s.

Feeding the Five Billion

How many people can the world feed? This question is central to the future of the planet Earth and its inhabitants. It is difficult enough to feed the world now, let alone an increasing world population. Advances in twentieth-century medicine, including mass vaccination, insect control, sanitation, and the development of life-saving drugs such as antibiotics, have caused the death rate to plummet. It is estimated that the world reached its first billion people in around 1830. The world's second billion people were added by 1930, the third by 1960, and the fourth by 1975. Robert McNamara, during his presidency of the World Bank, summed it up in 1978 when he said: "Short of nuclear war itself, population growth is the greatest issue that the world faces over the decade ahead." By 1985, the world population totaled somewhere around 4.8 billion people.

Steady exponential population growth could suddenly exhaust the world's mineral wealth and food supplies. An old riddle shows how little time there may be for new technologies and ideas to help alleviate the problem. Imagine a pond in which a water lily is growing. The lily plant doubles its size each day. Growing unchecked, it will completely cover the pond in thirty days, choking off all other life. Since the plant appears to be small for so long, you decide not to cut it back until it covers half the pond. On what day must you finally take action? On day twenty-nine, with only one day to go before the deadline.

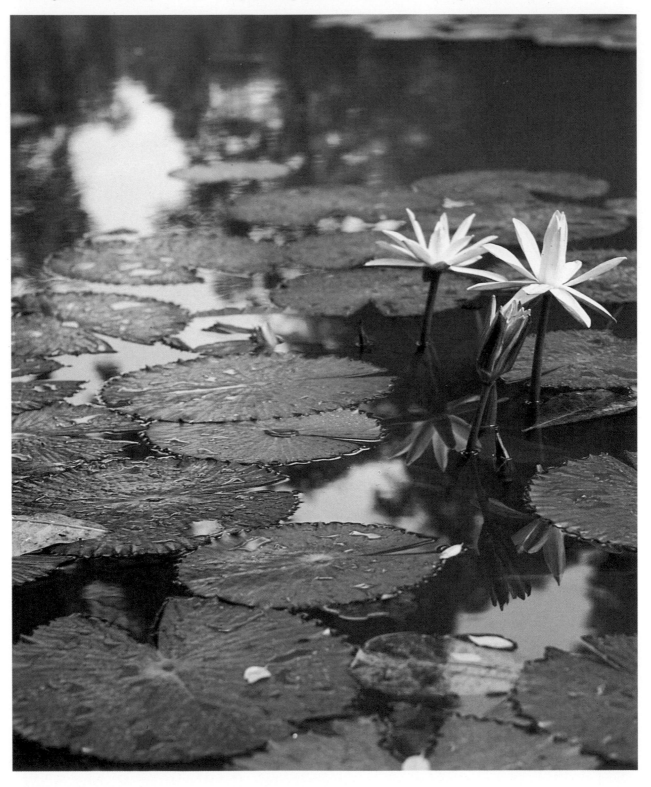

the expansion of its economy and the growth of its population in equilibrium.

A prediction in *The Resourceful Earth* — a book published in 1984 and written by a number of distinguished authors in response to the somewhat pessimistic outlook of *Global 2000* — is that although there will be more people on earth in the year 2000 it will not be more "crowded." The book predicts that "as the world's people have increasingly higher incomes, they will purchase better housing and mobility."

In LDCs, however, the emphasis is turning toward better population control in addition to economic development. If the birth–death equilibrium levels are reached by the turn of the century — that is, if the overall birth rate does not exceed the death rate — then the world population would stabilize at around 8.5 billion. If this stability is not reached until the year 2020 or 2025, then the "stable" figure is likely to be as much as 11 billion.

Many countries are striving to reduce their birth rates. China has implemented a number of stringent birth-control policies in its attempt to achieve zero population growth by the year 2000. The universal availability of contraception and the reward of high economic benefits to families having only one child have been a great success; since 1970 there has been a drop of thirty-four per cent in the birth rate. In Bangladesh, mothers and wives are regularly visited by local health workers who try to reduce the birth rate by providing various forms of contraception. Egypt pays a cash reward to women who are fitted with contraceptive IUDs, whereas in Thailand the fourth and subsequent children of a family miss out on welfare and educational benefits.

Aid to Africa

Although a number of countries have focused attention on the need for population control, some African countries have interpreted the developed world's insistence on birth control as subtle genocide. Others regard it as a reluctance of the rich nations to share their wealth and resources with the poor. The International Planned Parenthood Federation (IPPF), an organization pledged to increase public and government awareness of the

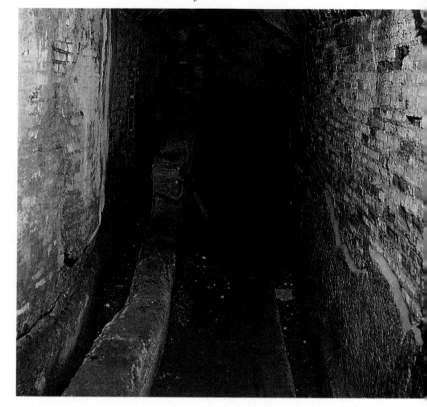

In towns and cities, the safe disposal of sewage is an obvious necessity for public health. This fact was acknowledged by the Romans, when they constructed this sewer beneath an Italian city.

interrelationship between population, development and resources, firmly believes in family planning. According to its secretary-general, Dr. Carl Wahren: "Fertility regulation alone does not solve socioeconomic problems but it has been conclusively shown that family planning contributes substantially to individual, family and community well-being."

The IPPF stresses that governments must try to make available the more widely acceptable techniques of contraception. It also emphasizes the need also to pay greater attention to population education and to improve the delivery of family planning services.

An underlying problem which the reduction of family size poses is the fear of people in LDCs that they will have nobody to look after them in their old age. With no health insurance or pension to protect them in a poor economy, the best investment strategy in such nations as India has, until now, been to produce many children. This is done in the hope that some of them will be able to

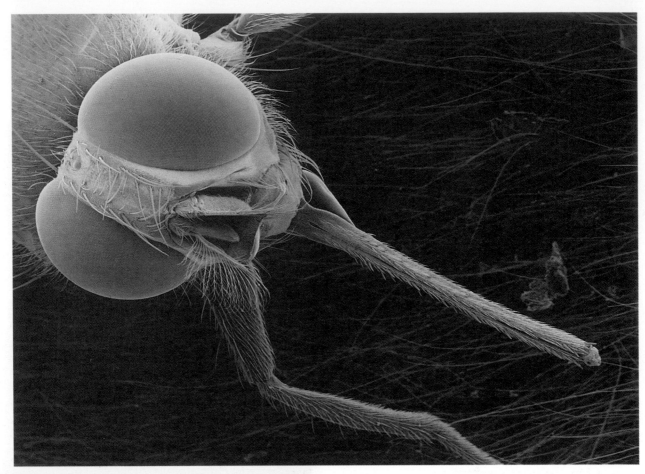

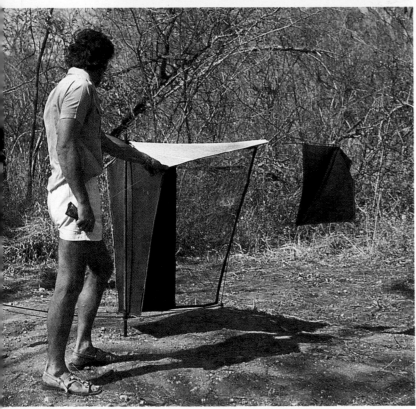

Resembling an armored invader from outer space, a tsetse fly (above) prepares to suck the blood of its human host. The tsetse fly transmits a parasitic protozoan which causes sleeping sickness in humans, and a deadly disease called nagana in cattle and horses. In one attempt to kill this parasite, radiation was used to sterilize male flies, making them unable to reproduce. Despite its primitive appearance, the tsetse fly-trap (bottom) has proved by far the most effective method of extermination. The flies are lured by jars containing chemicals extracted from cattle to a black cloth impregnated with insecticide, which kills them.

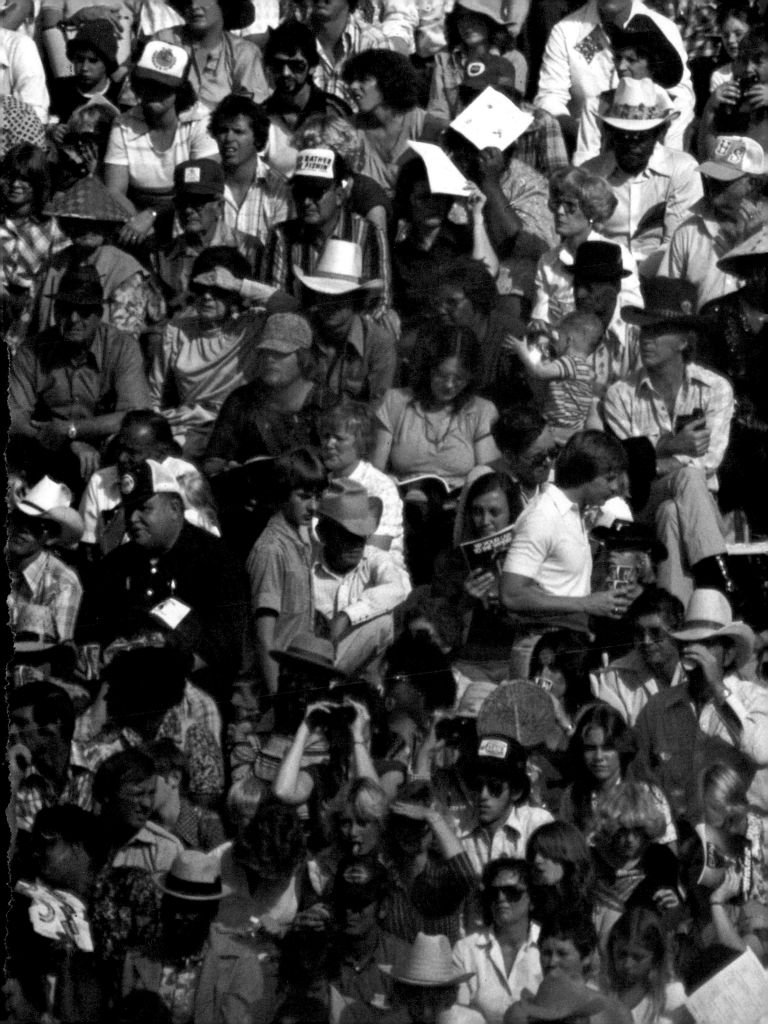

The future health and well-being of the people of the world can be encapsulated in three statistics: birth rate (expressed as the number of births per thousand population), population density (persons per square mile) and life expectancy (in years). Charted here are the figures for a range of typical countries for 1985 and demographic predictions for the situation forty years later, in the year 2025. In highly developed nations, such as the United States, Canada, the United Kingdom, the Soviet Union, Japan and Australia, there should be little change except a slight fall in birth rate and a small increase in life expectancy.

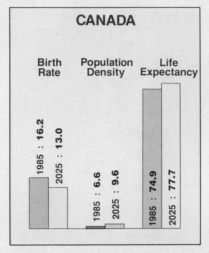

UNITED STATES

Birth Rate — 1985 : 16.0 — 2025 : 13.6
Population Density — 1985 : 65.2 — 2025 : 97.7
Life Expectancy — 1985 : 74.0 — 2025 : 77.4

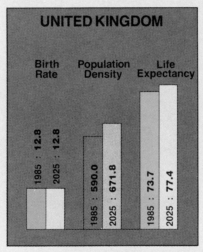

CANADA

Birth Rate — 1985 : 16.2 — 2025 : 13.0
Population Density — 1985 : 6.6 — 2025 : 9.6
Life Expectancy — 1985 : 74.9 — 2025 : 77.7

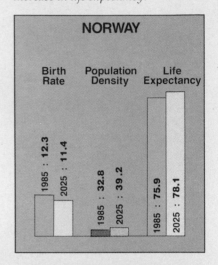

NORWAY

Birth Rate — 1985 : 12.3 — 2025 : 11.4
Population Density — 1985 : 32.8 — 2025 : 39.2
Life Expectancy — 1985 : 75.9 — 2025 : 78.1

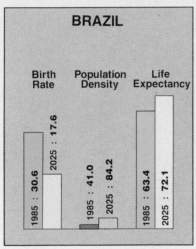

BRAZIL

Birth Rate — 1985 : 30.6 — 2025 : 17.6
Population Density — 1985 : 41.0 — 2025 : 84.2
Life Expectancy — 1985 : 63.4 — 2025 : 72.1

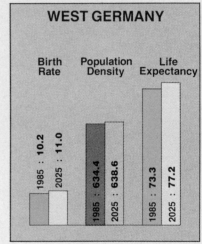

UNITED KINGDOM

Birth Rate — 1985 : 12.8 — 2025 : 12.8
Population Density — 1985 : 590.0 — 2025 : 671.8
Life Expectancy — 1985 : 73.7 — 2025 : 77.4

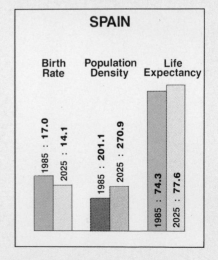

WEST GERMANY

Birth Rate — 1985 : 10.2 — 2025 : 11.0
Population Density — 1985 : 634.4 — 2025 : 638.6
Life Expectancy — 1985 : 73.3 — 2025 : 77.2

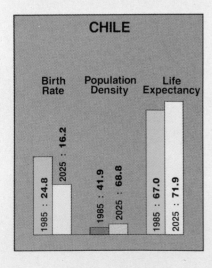

CHILE

Birth Rate — 1985 : 24.8 — 2025 : 16.2
Population Density — 1985 : 41.9 — 2025 : 68.8
Life Expectancy — 1985 : 67.0 — 2025 : 71.9

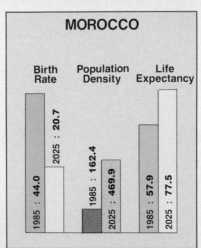

MOROCCO

Birth Rate — 1985 : 44.0 — 2025 : 20.7
Population Density — 1985 : 162.4 — 2025 : 469.9
Life Expectancy — 1985 : 57.9 — 2025 : 77.5

SPAIN

Birth Rate — 1985 : 17.0 — 2025 : 14.1
Population Density — 1985 : 201.1 — 2025 : 270.9
Life Expectancy — 1985 : 74.3 — 2025 : 77.6

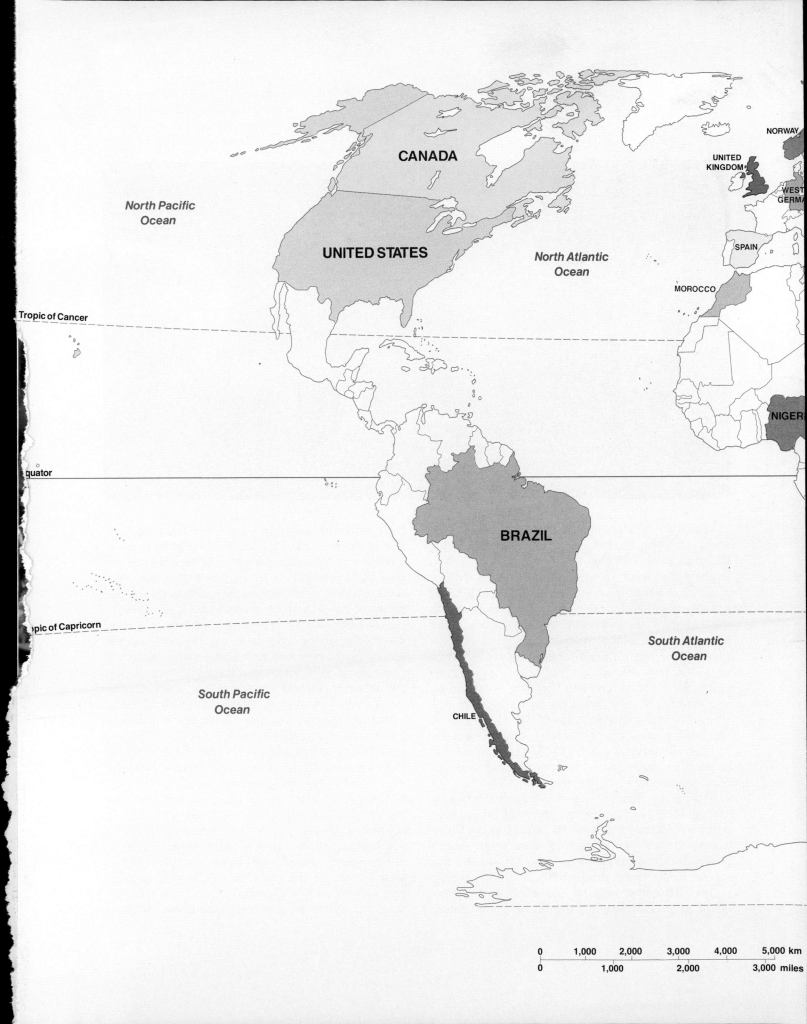

CANADA

North Pacific
Ocean

UNITED STATES

North Atlantic
Ocean

NORWAY

UNITED
KINGDOM

WEST
GERMA

SPAIN

MOROCCO

NIGER

Tropic of Cancer

Equator

BRAZIL

Tropic of Capricorn

South Atlantic
Ocean

South Pacific
Ocean

CHILE

| 0 | 1,000 | 2,000 | 3,000 | 4,000 | 5,000 km |
| 0 | | 1,000 | | 2,000 | 3,000 miles |

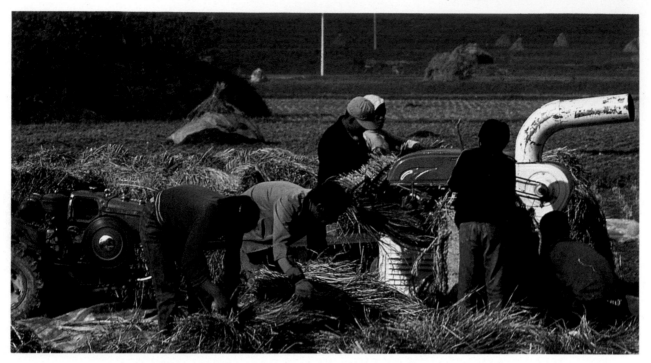

These converted tractors used for threshing rice may seem primitive in comparison to modern Western farming methods, but intermediate technology is often more appropriate for local rural communities.

provide care for their elderly parents, a "life insurance" attitude that has proved self-destructive for the country as a whole.

There has been considerable Western aid for health and malnutrition problems in the LDCs, yet massive famine still exists. The consensus among the experts in the international aid agencies is that economic policies are to blame. African governments have been accused of neglecting subsistence agriculture by devoting their best land to cash crops for export, and for holding food prices artificially low. The result is that people in the cities live on grain subsidized by aid budgets, while the rural poor try to scratch a living from the remaining marginal land. The Africans argue that colonialism trapped their economies into dependence on one or two cash crops.

African governments are becoming increasingly aware of the need for change, yet most attempts to develop Africa's rural areas have failed. Many experts believe that African governments should be developing enterprises for the small farmer who wants to increase productivity without getting bigger. The best aid the industrialized nations could give is in helping the farmers to develop their agricultural systems on a low-technology or intermediate-technology basis. There is no point in having a sophisticated high-tech harvester if the crop yield is small. It would seem that the solutions to long-term famine are ultimately in the hands of the African farmers themselves.

Low technology is also important for controlling disease in Africa. Scientists are encouraging the use of local resources and skills, rather than the purchase of equipment and importation of expertise from developed countries. For instance, the tsetse fly has always caused enormous problems to African farmers as a carrier of sleeping sickness in humans and a similar disease in animals. So far, attempts at controlling the fly have failed. A new technique which is cheap and simple is being developed by British scientists.

A sheet of black cloth impregnated with the insecticide pyrethrin is stretched on wire frames; beneath it, on the ground, are placed jars containing small quantities of chemicals, extracted from cattle, which attract the tsetse fly. Acetone is added to make the chemicals evaporate quickly. The flies swarm to the screens and are killed as they attempt to suck blood from them. Tests in

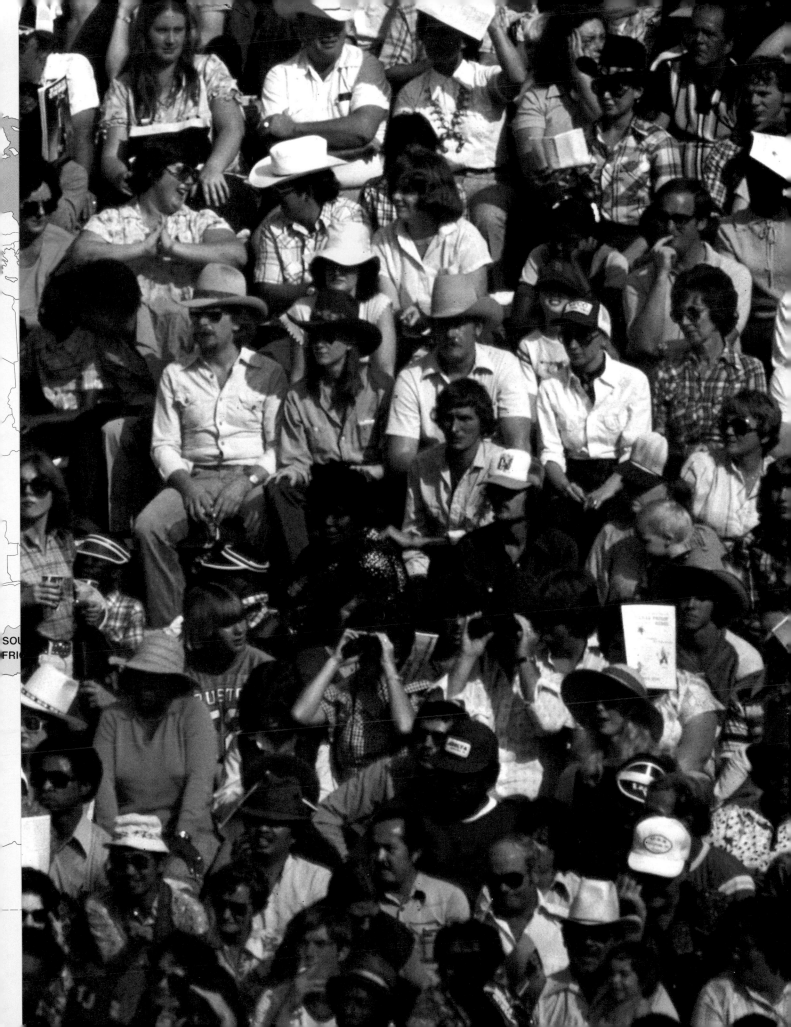

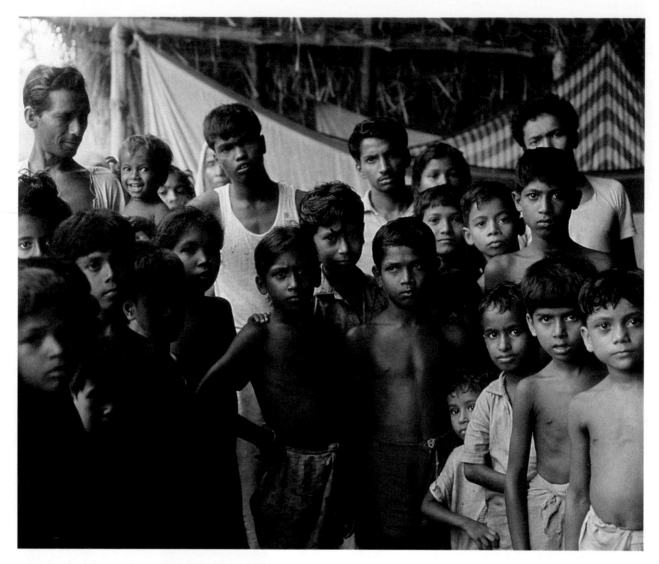

Zimbabwe have shown this to be a highly successful method, much better than the comparatively expensive and wasteful procedure of ground spraying. By using other attractant chemicals which are currently being developed, the technique should eventually become more effective and even cheaper.

Intimations of Immortality

At the beginning of this century, life expectancy in the United States was only forty-seven years. In 1985 it was just over seventy years for males, and seventy-eight years for females. One of the consequences of improved health care, particularly in the developed nations, is that populations now contain increasing numbers of elderly people. The problems of old age on a large scale are relatively new, and have existed only since people learned to overcome the environment well enough to live beyond their reproductive years.

Conquering disease by advances in hygiene and medicine have been major keys to the increase in the proportion of the elderly. As more is learned about the nature of disease — particularly cancer — then this figure can be expected to increase. Although scientists have been able to increase life expectancy, none has made any significant progress in extending the maximum life span. This is despite considerable research into the theories and processes of aging, particularly that carried out in the United States.

The maximum age reached by the longest surviving individuals since the Romans first started keeping records is between 110 and 120 years. Because maximum life span is statistically predictable, scientists in general think that aging is not just related to wear and tear, or there would be some "well preserved people" who would live to be older than 120. Intrinsic factors thus seem to hold the key to aging — factors that are thought to

In countries such as India, large families (left) traditionally provide help for parents in the event of illness, particularly during old age. In this way, the numerous children act as a kind of health insurance.

More people create a need for more living space. This monk seal is one of thousands of species which, because of the need for land by the world's rapidly increasing population, face the threat of extinction.

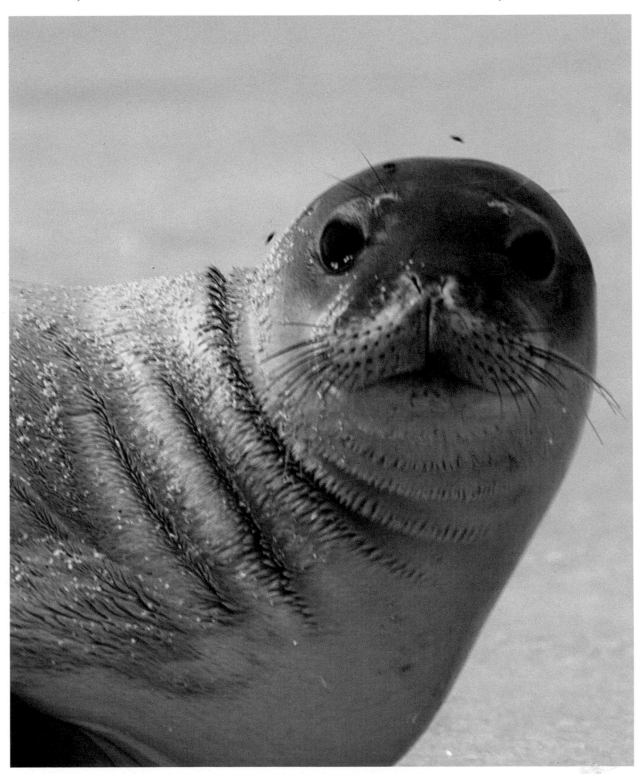

Carl Rogers

Patient Understanding

During the twentieth century the importance of mental health to human well-being has become much better understood. In the past, the mentally ill were shut away in conditions of harsh imprisonment, or put on public display for popular amusement. Psychiatry in the 1980s seeks to comfort and heal.

The work of many influential people has been fundamental to this change in attitude. High on the list, along with Sigmund Freud, the father of psychoanalysis, and B. F. Skinner, originator of the Behaviorist school of psychiatry, is Skinner's contemporary Carl Rogers, founder of the school of Humanistic Psychology.

Carl Ransom Rogers was born in January 1902 in Oak Park, Illinois. Educated locally, he began university by taking an agricultural course — his father owned a farm — but then switched to history. On graduation, however, he joined a Protestant theological college in New York. After two years he decided he had no vocation toward a religious life, and thereupon enrolled for a postgraduate degree in clinical psychology. His master's degree came in 1928, and his doctorate in 1931, both from Columbia University.

Rogers' first work was for the

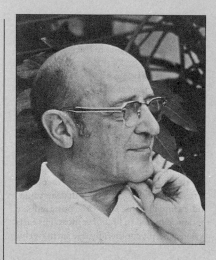

Society for the Prevention of Cruelty to Children child guidance center at Rochester, N.Y., where, after a few years, he became Director. From a lectureship at Rochester University he then became Professor of Clinical Psychology at Ohio State University in 1940, but in the meantime achieved some fame, through his writings, as an innovative therapist. As Professor of Psychology at the University of Chicago from 1945, Rogers helped to set up a counseling center, employing his methods and analyzing the results. From 1957 until his retirement he was Professor of Psychology and Psychiatry at the University of Wisconsin at Madison.

It may have been Rogers' original leanings toward the ministry that later made him specially aware of the innate humanity of each of his patients. Whereas other psychiatrists required a sort of teacher-pupil relationship with their patients in which the "teacher" took on a fairly dominant role and directed the treatment according to his or her understanding of the patient's progress, Rogers instead gave the psychiatrist a non-directive status. He let the patient (whom he called the "client") decide how progress was to be made: the psychiatrist was there as a friend, in a person-to-person role, to restate (without interpreting) the patient's own expressed words, desires and aspirations in such a way that the patient became aware of his or her motivations or repressions, and could change life style accordingly. This non-critical, catalystic attitude on the part of the therapist is a fundamental principle of Humanistic Psychology.

Another principle on which Rogers theorized was that of the integration of the Self — of the way in which we experience our lives and feelings, and of the way we perceive that others see us. To Rogers, such integration was the goal of all therapy. Late in life, Rogers became fascinated by group therapy, particularly as practiced among the developmental clinics in California.

be locked within the genetic material of human cells. One school of thought is that the state of aging is controlled by specific aging genes, collectively known as the "supergene," and it has been suggested by some American scientists that by genetically engineering the "supergene" and introducing it into humans, men and women will eventually be able to live longer.

Another theory is that there are a number of random errors which accumulate in the genetic material of the cell. As the errors build up during cell aging, the cell can no longer perform its allocated functions. If these "errors" could be reduced, we could live longer.

Yet another theory is that the body contains toxic by-products of oxygen metabolism known as free radicals. These are thought to damage or age cells. It is also thought that the body responds to free radicals by producing enzymes that act as antioxidants, searching out free radicals and combining with them before any real damage is done. As people get older, though, enzyme production decreases. To counter this, some American scientists have suggested that we should supplement our diet with antioxidants — substances that include vitamins C and E, and also selenium — to slow down aging.

The Californian gerontologist, Dr. Roy Walford, advocates taking doses of antioxidants in an attempt to postpone aging. He advises readers of his best-selling book *Maximum Life Span* to do the same. He is optimistic about halting or slowing aging and believes scientists will find out exactly how to do so before the year 2000. Dr. Walford, along with other scientists, has shown that the life spans of mice can be extended simply by limiting the amount of food they eat. He believes that a restricted diet would also reduce the incidence of cancer, kidney and heart disease in humans, just as it has in animals. To prove his point Dr. Walford now fasts two days a week and restricts himself to a diet that totals about 2,000 calories a day for the other five days.

Care for Senior Citizens

Since the proportion of elderly people in industrialized developed nations is increasing, so the number of problems in looking after old people

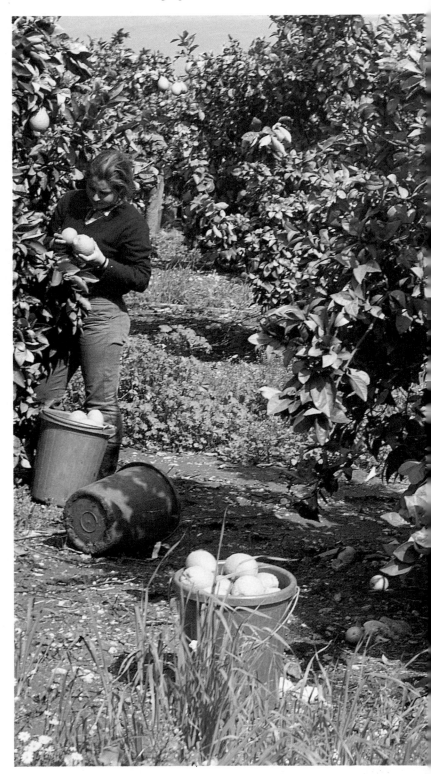

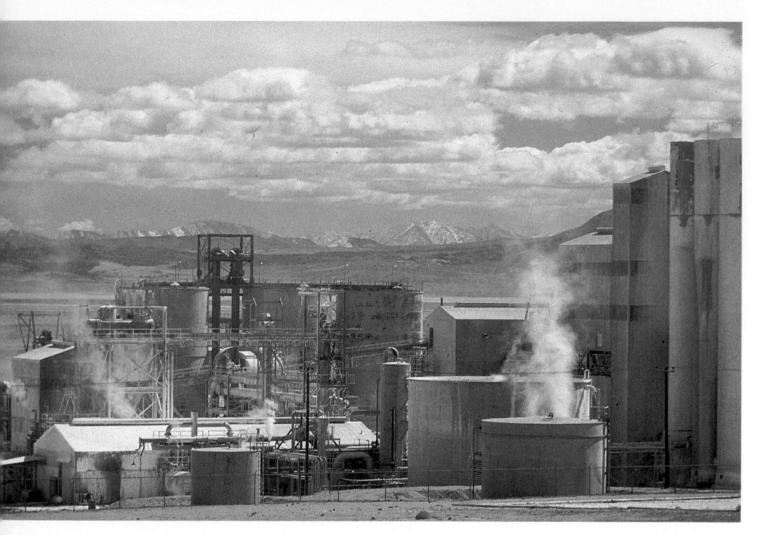

*One approach to a world food
shortage is to make synthetic food in a
chemical plant* (left). *An example is a
biochemical process for making
protein out of substances extracted
from petroleum. The synthetic
protein can be formed into fibers and
compressed to give the texture of
meat, and flavored to taste like
chicken, pork or beef.*

has increased also. In the future there will be many
more elderly people with the chronic diseases of
old age, and improved medical services will have
to be provided to postpone their mental and physical decline. Cardiovascular diseases, cancer,
mental disorders, arthritis and permanent disability are potentially the major health problems of the
elderly. Add to these the economic and social
difficulties that together can create a situation of
dependence, and the result is that caring for the
elderly will be an increasingly necessary and major
industry by the year 2000.

The proportion of the American population that
is sixty-five or older increased from four per cent in
1920 to more than eleven per cent by 1985. In 1900,
only thirty-seven per cent of infants born reached
sixty-five years of age. In 1985 more than seventy-
five per cent of infants could expect to live for
sixty-five years or more. This trend is similar in
other industrialized nations. In some poor countries, the proportion of people over sixty-five years
of age is as low as two or three per cent.

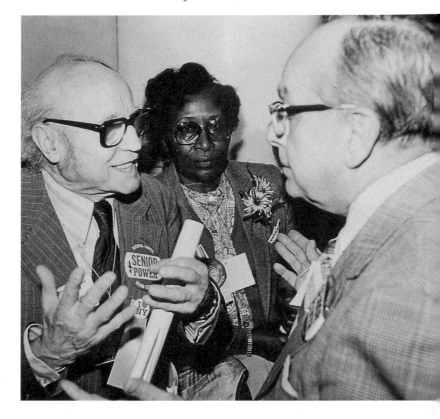

One staggering prediction is that by the year 2000 there will be a hundred thousand people in the United States aged more than one hundred. And presumably there will be many centenarians alive in other industrialized countries. It is already known that the human body can sustain life for more than a century, given a proper diet and the absence of serious illness. So advances in medical science, and the elimination of bad eating habits and smoking, together with the removal of hazards at the workplace and the home, should allow more and more people to live up to an age of a hundred years or so.

Another impact on survival is likely to come from a drastic reduction in the number of car accidents. It is predicted that by the year 2035 there will be only ten per cent of the accidents that occurred in 1985. Sweden is experimenting with microprocessor technology that would make this improvement possible, for example by the use of sensors buried in the road linked to on-board car computers.

The United States has to face the challenge of having an increased elderly population — and the signs are that it is doing so. Younger people are acknowledging the fact that they, too, will probably live to a very old age, and will probably retire younger than their parents, and are therefore preparing accordingly.

The Financial Burden

In the United States, the average economic status of people over sixty-five has steadily increased as a result of automatic annual Social Security cost-of-living adjustments since 1974, and increases in the number of persons receiving private pensions. Americans have realized the need to invest in their old age. Social Security is a major source of income for a substantial part of the aging population, so the future welfare of many Americans will depend upon Social Security levels set by the government.

One of the many problems faced by today's government is budgeting. A person who enrolled in January 1937, when Social Security started, and who since then has paid in the maximum contribution each year until January 1984, has paid in a total of $19,169. He or she would, in 1986, get that investment back within two to three years. Pre-

vious governments never expected that so many people would be around fifty years on, nor that there would be such a drain on national funds. In 1982, according to the Office of Management and Budget estimate, benefits to the aged accounted for some twenty-seven per cent of the entire Federal budget. It has been projected that without any further liberalization, demographic developments alone are likely to increase the percentage of the Federal budget spent on the elderly to thirty-five per cent by the year 2000 and sixty-five per cent by the year 2050.

Government agencies have also predicted that by the year 2000 there will only be three workers for every beneficiary, compared to around 3.3 per beneficiary in 1985. By the year 2025, the ratio is expected to drop to two to one. The slower growth in the younger segment of the population, because of the falling birth rate, will also mean that fewer active workers will be making payments into public and private pension programs, whereas a greater number of older workers will be eligi-

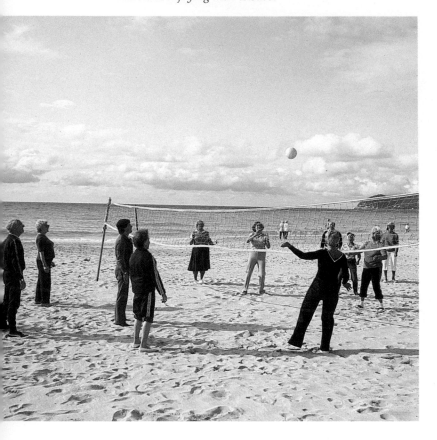

Center for Health Statistics estimates that, by the year 2000, people aged sixty-five or more will be responsible for thirty-eight per cent of the 331 million days of short-stay hospital care projected for the population as a whole (an increase of twenty-six per cent). They will also comprise seventeen per cent of all visits to physicians' offices (an increase of twenty-two per cent).

As in the provision of social security benefits, the flow of resources into such areas will have to increase to cope with the aging population. Policy on aging, which involves political competition between many interest groups, has one major asset: the aged are the one minority to which everyone anticipates belonging. Investment in care for the elderly is thus an investment in the future of mankind. The same is true whether the money is spent on improving health care in hospitals, or on providing supplementary support for the care of the elderly at home.

The need for an increase in government-provided services for the elderly depends, in part, on the fact that families are smaller and aging parents cannot rely on their children for support. In 1931, nearly one-half of all women aged between sixty and sixty-four had had four or more children. By 1980, the proportion had dropped to one in four. Although the over-eighties are a group with relatively large numbers of children (reflecting the high birth rates of the past), the 1980s are expected to show a sharp increase in the percentage of older women with small families. The 1990s are expected to see a brief reversal of the trend as a reflection of the postwar "baby boom."

Although a large number of elderly people need family or state care, there are also many able to lead an active life, particularly those who have retired in their sixties or earlier. The trend has been toward an increase in the average level of educational attainment of old people, and their involvement in cultural activities is expected to increase. Whether there is a significant increase in cultural facilities for the elderly will depend on how many activities are provided, and on their accessibility and price. Travel is the major leisure-time activity for retired elderly Americans, and a growth in the travel industry can be expected in order to cater to the ever increasing need.

ble to draw pension benefits. The United States government is therefore keen to increase employment opportunities for the elderly for fiscal and economic reasons.

When people do choose to retire, and where they decide to live, often depends upon their personal fitness or the ability of their families or the nation to look after them. The nursing-home population increased dramatically from 505,000 individuals in nursing homes in 1963 to around one and a half million in 1985. Most of these people are aged sixty-five or older. It seems likely, therefore, that greater government and private expenditure will be needed to expand the number of nursing homes to accommodate the increasing need. The number of nursing-home residents in the year 2000 is expected to be almost two million, assuming current rates of growth.

Nursing-home utilization is thus expected to be the fastest-growing segment of the health care system in the next two decades. The National

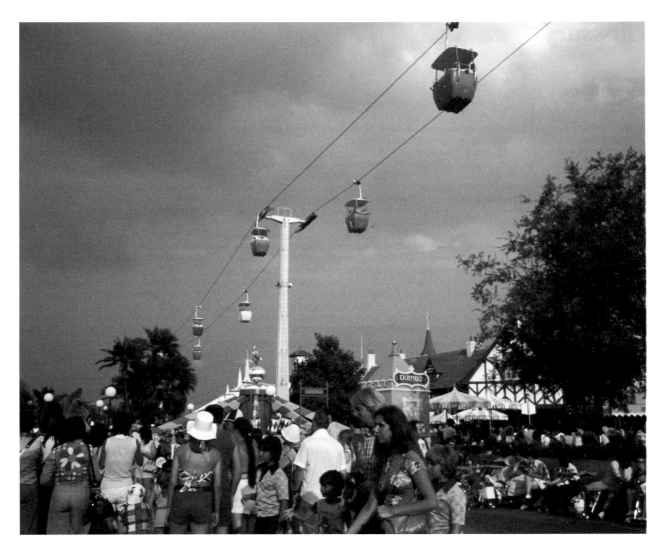

Sport and physical exercise are also popular among the elderly. While elderly people cannot be expected to play sports such as baseball, an entrepreneurial expansion will probably take place toward activities they might reasonably participate in, such as swimming, golf and tennis. A survey in 1977 showed that nearly half of all persons aged sixty-five or more followed a regular exercise regime. The shape of sports facilities might thus be expected to change dramatically toward pursuits for the elderly as the year 2000 approaches.

Medicine's future is closely linked with that of humanity. The advances in science and technology that allow physicians to understand, and so prevent and treat, illness can greatly improve human life and social well-being. But the effectiveness with which these advances are used is dependent on the social values, and on the political decisions, that determine their allocation. All of us, thus, have a role to play in deciding how medical advances will alter the future.

Happy and optimistic, many thousands of American families every year revel in the delights of Walt Disney World. The ability to relax is an essential ingredient contributing to a long healthy life. Now that advances are being made in medical and health care, coupled with increasingly positive attitudes to the problems of aging, old age may well be pushed further into the future for most of us who are alive today. The prospects for a happier and healthier, as well as a longer, life are excellent.

histocompatibility antigen a protein on a cell surface that forms a complex with the protein of an invading virus.

homeopathic therapy a technique of alternative medical treatment which use minute amounts of a drug that in a healthy person would cause symptoms of the disease.

hyperactivity abnormally high levels of activity.

hypnosis the induction of an artificial sleep or a trance-like state under which the subject is highly suggestible and acts only when directed to do so.

immune systems those systems in the body that act to repel invasion by "foreign" organisms and tissues.

immunology the study of the body's resistance to infection and "foreign" tissues.

immunosuppressive describes a substance that stops or reduces the action of the immune system.

in vitro in a test tube and laboratory, as opposed to in a living organism.

inhibitor something that stops or slows down a process or action.

insulin a hormone produced by the islets of Langerhans in the pancreas, and important in regulating blood sugars such as glucose.

insulin pump a device designed to give a metered dose of insulin, at regular intervals, to people with diabetes mellitus.

intravenous within a vein, as with the injection of some drugs or fluids.

larynx the voice box, made up of nine cartilages and enclosing the vocal cords.

leprosy a chronic bacterial disease in which the skin thickens and ulcerates and there is a loss of sensation.

leukemia a cancer of the blood-forming tissue, characterized by excessive numbers of white blood cells.

local anesthetic a substance with the property of removing sensation from the area to which it is applied but not from the rest of the body.

lymphocytes white blood cells which have an important role in producing antibodies to infection.

magnetic resonance spectroscopy a technique for building up a picture of the inside of the body by detecting the differential "resonance" of separate areas of tissue to the passage of electromagnetic waves.

maladaptation failure to adapt to the needs imposed by the surroundings.

malignant describes a type of cancer in which growth spreads into surrounding tissue or gives rise to secondary tumors in other parts of the body.

malnutrition a condition in which the body does not receive food in either sufficient quantity or quality for the maintenance of health.

marker a length of DNA with a particular composition that always occurs in subjects with a certain characteristic or defect. The specific gene for the characteristic might be expected to occur within the marker segment.

microbiology the study of microscopic organisms.

microsurgery techniques for carrying out operations on a microscopic scale, down to the level of a single cell.

monoclonal antibodies artificially manufactured antibodies made to combat a specific target.

monocyte a white blood cell with a single nucleus. Most monocytes occur in the spleen and liver, where they destroy foreign bodies and old red cells.

MS multiple sclerosis.

multiple sclerosis a degenerative disease of the brain and spinal cord, resulting in various types of paralysis and lack of coordination.

muscular dystrophy an inherited disease in which there is progressive degeneration of the muscles.

mutation a change in a gene or genes that occurs apparently spontaneously or as a result of outside influences; an organism formed from a reproductive

cell in which such a change has occurred.

neonatal born recently.

neurotransmitter any substance produced at nerve endings that transmits a signal from one nerve cell to the next.

NMR nuclear magnetic resonance.

nuclear magnetic resonance (NMR) the differential "resonance" of different parts of the body to electromagnetic radiation.

obstetrician a medical practitioner who specializes in the care of women before, during and just after giving birth.

occlusion blockage of a passage or a blood vessel.

oncogenes genes implicated in causing cancer.

open surgery any surgery that involves opening up the body.

orthopedist a medical practitioner specializing in injuries and disorders of bones and joints.

oscillatory moving backward and forward.

osteoarthritis a disorder of the joints in which the cartilage layers covering the ends of the bones at the joint, and sometimes the bones themselves, are gradually worn away.

ovulation the release of an egg from an ovary.

Parkinson's disease, or Parkinsonism a degenerative disease of the nervous system, characterized by a gross tremor of the hands and muscular rigidity.

pasteurization a technique for killing bacteria in milk, wine and other liquids by heating to about 150°F.

pathology the study of the causes and nature of disease, and the changes in the body brought about by it.

PCB polychlorinated biphenyl.

pharmacopeia originally a book listing drugs and their uses; also used to describe the range of drugs available to medicine.

photochemical smog   a chemical pall hanging over cities in some types of climate, in which the components include toxic chemicals produced by the effects of light on simple molecules.

physiological   dealing with the functions of the body rather than its anatomy.

pinna   the external ear, the flap of skin and cartilage surrounding the orifice of the ear.

platelets   small particles in the blood which play an important part in the blood clotting mechanism.

polychlorinated biphenyls   a class of synthetic organic chemicals which are known carcinogens and pollutants.

presenile dementia   Alzheimer's disease.

prophylactic   tending to prevent or protect against an effect or disorder.

prosthesis   an artificial substitute for part of the body, such as an artificial limb.

psychiatry   treatments and therapies to counter disorders of the mind.

psychosomatic   describing illness that is wholly or partly attributable to mental factors, even though there are physical symptoms.

psychotherapy   treatment of a disorder — particularly a behavioral disorder — by attempting to improve the mental condition, rather than treat the physical symptoms.

puerperal   of, or caused by, childbirth.

pulmonary   of the lung.

pustule   a small raised bump on the skin containing pus; a pimple.

radiography   the use of X rays or other penetrating radiation to produce an image on a screen or photographic film.

renal   of the kidney.

replication   the process of making an exact copy, especially of cells or DNA.

reprogram   produce a new set of instructions for functioning.

schizophrenia   a group of various mental illnesses in which the sufferer may have delusions, may have difficulty recognizing the real from the imagined, and may not connect thought and action.

sepsis   poisoning of the body tissues by invading bacteria.

septicemia   blood-poisoning by bacteria.

sickle-cell anemia   a hereditary disease in which the red blood cells assume a thin sickle shape.

sleeping sickness   a disease caused by the single-celled organism *Trypanosoma*, with symptoms that include fever and extreme lethargy. It is transmitted by the tsetse fly.

stroke   a seizure, and any resulting paralysis, caused by a blood clot in one of the brain's arteries.

substance P   a substance released by nerves that is concerned in the perception of pain.

suppressor cell   a type of white blood cell believed to be involved in recognizing the body's own tissues and stopping any immune response to them.

syphilis   a bacterial disease spread by sexual contact which, if untreated, leads by progressively more serious stages to death.

testosterone   a male sex hormone produced in the testes and responsible for the development of the male secondary sexual characteristics such as deep voice and facial hair.

thrombosis   a blood clot.

tissue plasminogen activator (tPa)   an enzyme with the property of dissolving red blood cells away from a blood clot.

tissue-typed   describes a tissue which has been matched to one with standard known characteristics.

TNF   tumor necrosis factor.

tPa   tissue plasminogen activator.

transfection   the process by which segments of "foreign" DNA are mixed with cells to make them assimilate the DNA into their own genetic material.

transgenic   describes an organism that has incorporated in it genetic material from an outside source.

transplantation   the transfer of organs or tissue from one organism to another.

tsetse fly   a fly of the genus *Glossina* that occurs in parts of Africa. It is the carrier of sleeping sickness.

tuberculosis   a bacterial disease in which nodules form in the tissues, especially the lungs, and there may be fever and wasting.

tumor necrosis factor (TNF)   a protein produced by white blood cells of the single-nucleus type, which has the property of destroying some types of cancer cell.

typhus   a disease caused by the microorganism *Rickettsia*, and transmitted by fleas and lice. Symptoms include skin eruptions and fever.

urethral   of the urethra, the tube that carries urine from the bladder to the outside of the body.

urology   the study of disorders of the urinary system.

vaccination   the introduction, commonly by injection, of a vaccine to induce immunity.

vaccine   a preparation of a virus which has been killed by heat treatment or weakened so that it is no longer a threat. It is so named because the first such preparation was made of cowpox (*Vaccinia*) virus and was used to combat the similar smallpox virus.

vascular   of the blood vessels.

ventilation   the movement of air into and out of the lungs, usually applied to a machine for this purpose.

virus   a type of minute organism which can survive only by invading a cell in another organism, taking control of some of the cell's activities and reproducing itself. Outside a host a virus appears inert and lifeless. Many human diseases are caused by viruses.

Illustration Credits

Index

Some time ago, in a land you'll never find on a map, lived a boy named Jack and a mom named Mom. They shared a small house and a sad, empty garden.

"I'm so hungry, I could eat my shoes," Jack said.

"I'm hungry too," Mom said. "I'd make a dirt sandwich, but we're out of bread."

One afternoon, Jack looked out the window at their bony cow named Gloria. She mooed and ate the last pea in the garden. Jack's stomach rumbled.

"We have to do something," he told Mom, "or we're going to starve!"

Gloria stuck out her tongue and swished her tail.

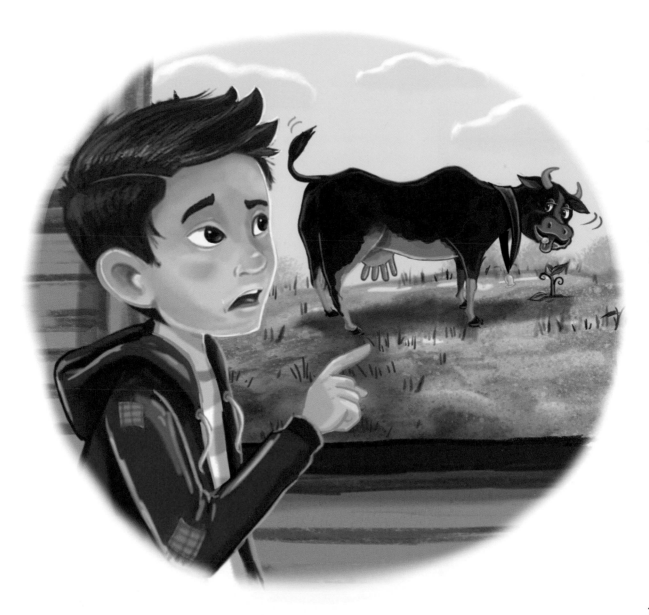

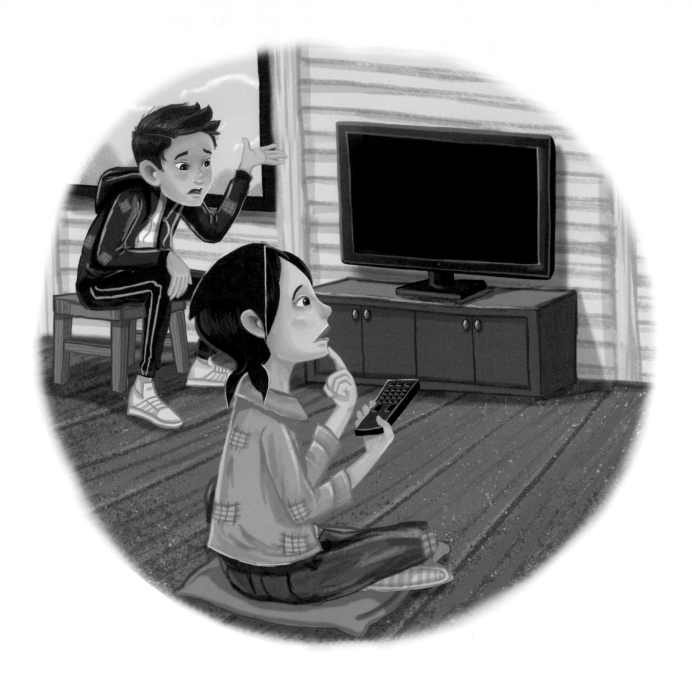

"That's it," Jack said. "I'm going to town to sell that awful cow!"

"Good idea," Mom said, staring at the blank TV screen. "Then we can pay our cable bill."

Jack groaned. "No, we need to buy *food*, Mom."

"Oh, of course," she replied. "Sorry."

Jack went outside, grabbed Gloria's rope, and pulled. The cow wouldn't budge.

"Moo," she said.

"How about you *moo-ve* instead?" Jack said.

"How's it going, Jack?" Mom called from the window.

"I'm pulling on the rope, using a force, but this annoying cow is just standing here," Jack replied.

"A force can be a pull *or* a push," Mom said. "Try pushing her. She'll move."

Jack pushed Gloria as hard as he could. With a grunt, she finally moved, and the two headed to town.

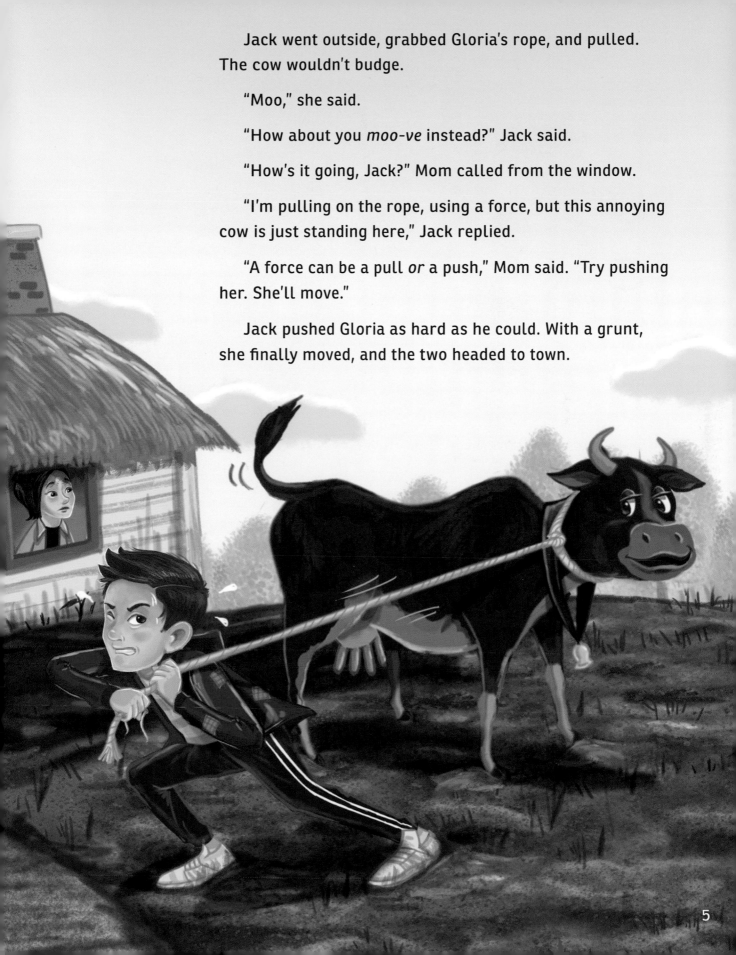

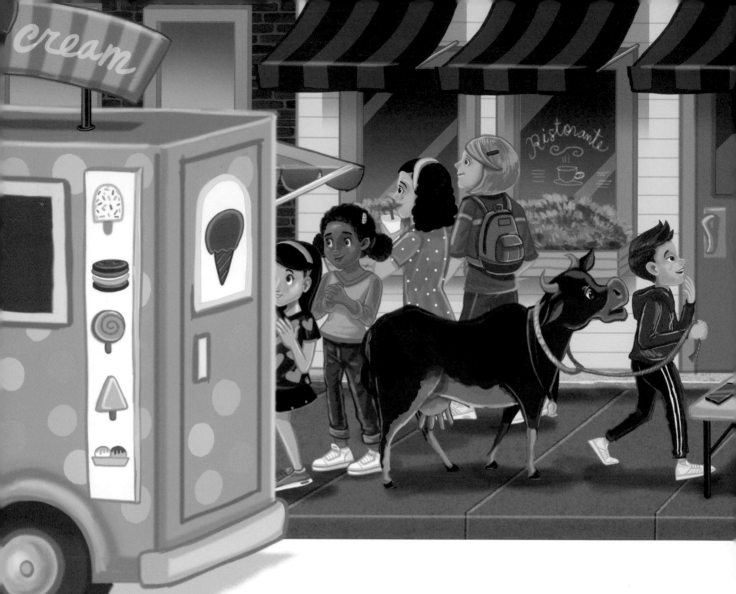

In town, people crowded the streets. They hurried from place to place. Not one of them wanted to buy a bony cow.

"Moo," Gloria said.

"Yeah, we need *moo-ney*," Jack said. "For food. And cable TV."

Just as Jack was ready to give up, he spotted a man selling cell phones and beans. Jack accidentally bumped into the man's table, and some beans fell onto the sidewalk.

"Oops," Jack said. "Sorry about that."

"No problem," the man said. "That's what gravity does!"

"Gravy?" Jack asked. "That sounds delicious right now."

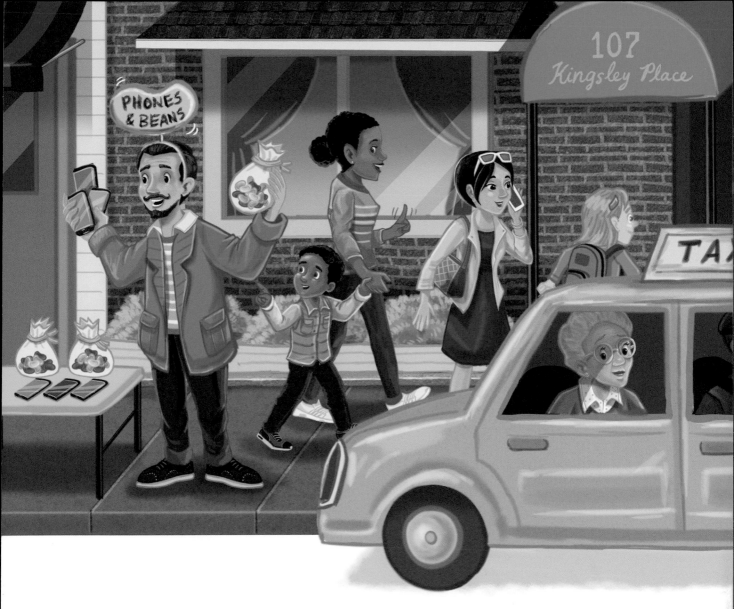

"No," the man said. "Not gravy, *gravity.* It's the force that pulls everything with mass toward Earth's center. Buildings, cars, people . . ."

"I thought things just fell," Jack said.

"*Gravity* makes that happen," the man explained. "Hey, would you like to trade me your cow for these beans?"

"I don't like beans," Jack said.

"Oh, but these are *magic* beans," the man said. "Plant them and you'll grow one amazing, giant-sized—"

"Yeah, OK, sure," Jack said.

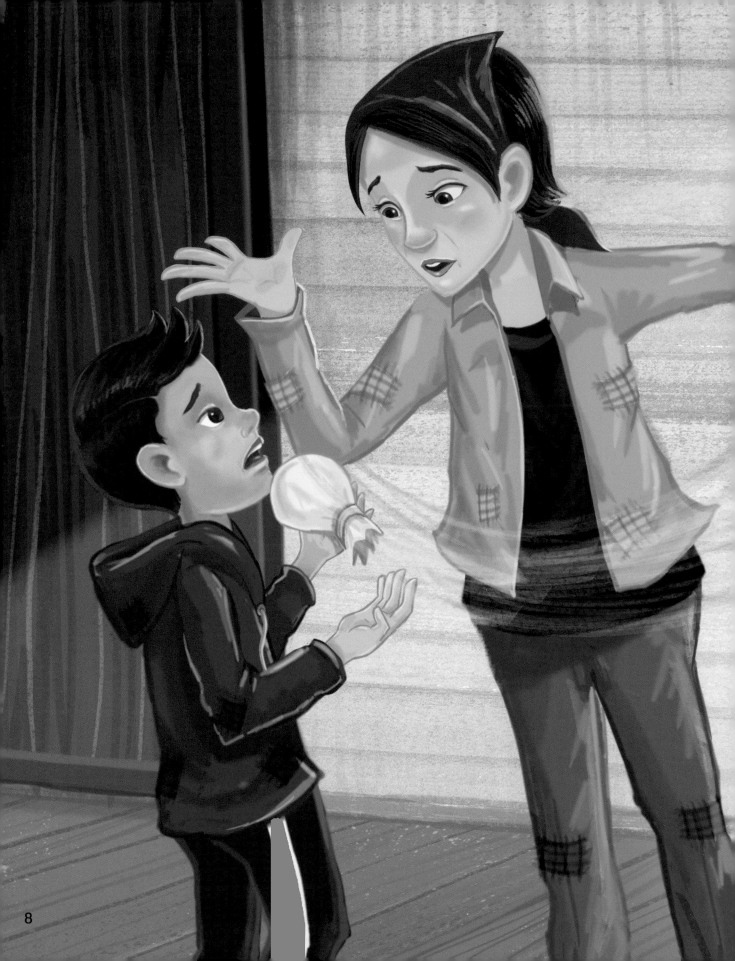

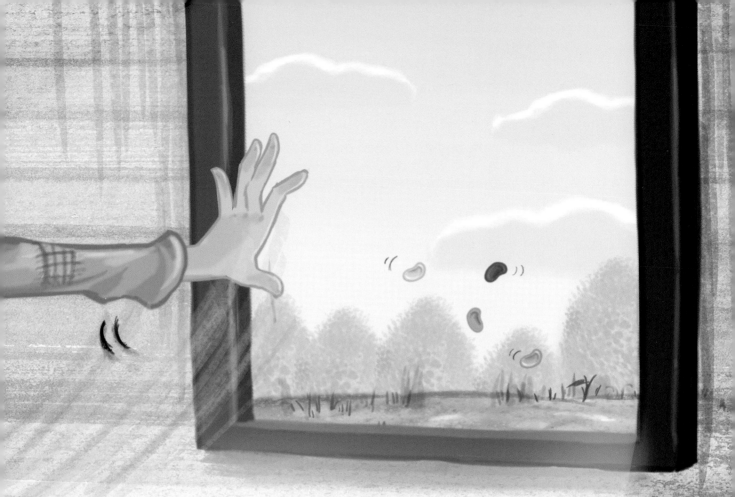

Jack couldn't wait to tell his mom the good news.

"Mom! Look!" Jack cried. "I got some beans!"

"We don't like beans," Mom said. "How much money did you get for the cow?"

"No money," Jack said. "Just these beans. *Magic* beans."

"Jack, beans only grow more beans," Mom said. She snatched them from her son's hand and threw them out the window. Hard. The tiny veggies disappeared in the garden dirt.

"Good arm, Mom," Jack said.

"Thank you," Mom said. "That *was* a lot of force, wasn't it?"

Late that night, a thunderstorm soaked the land with rain—and something happened in the garden.

"What is *that*?" Jack cried, looking out the window the next morning. He leapt from bed and raced outside. Mom followed.

A huge, thick beanstalk towered overhead. It stretched high into the clouds.

"Great," Mom said. "Now we'll have tons of giant beans we won't eat."

"I'll try to shake some loose," Jack said. He pushed on the beanstalk . . . and then pushed harder.

The beanstalk wouldn't budge.

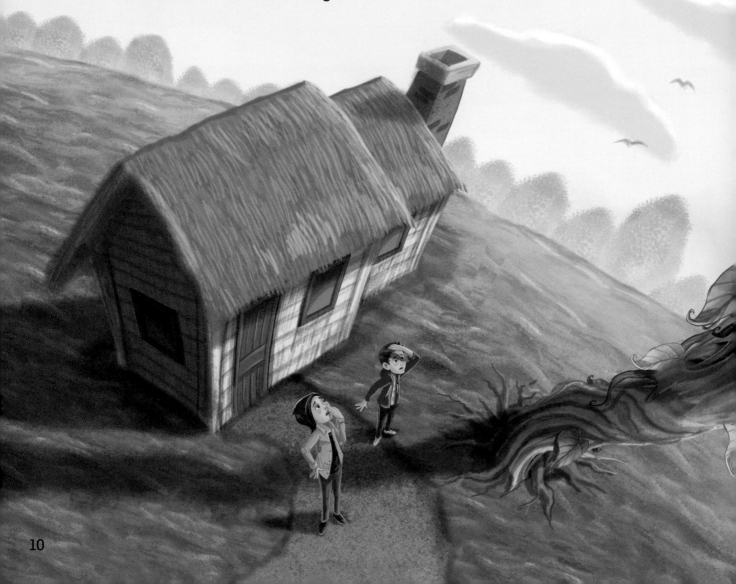

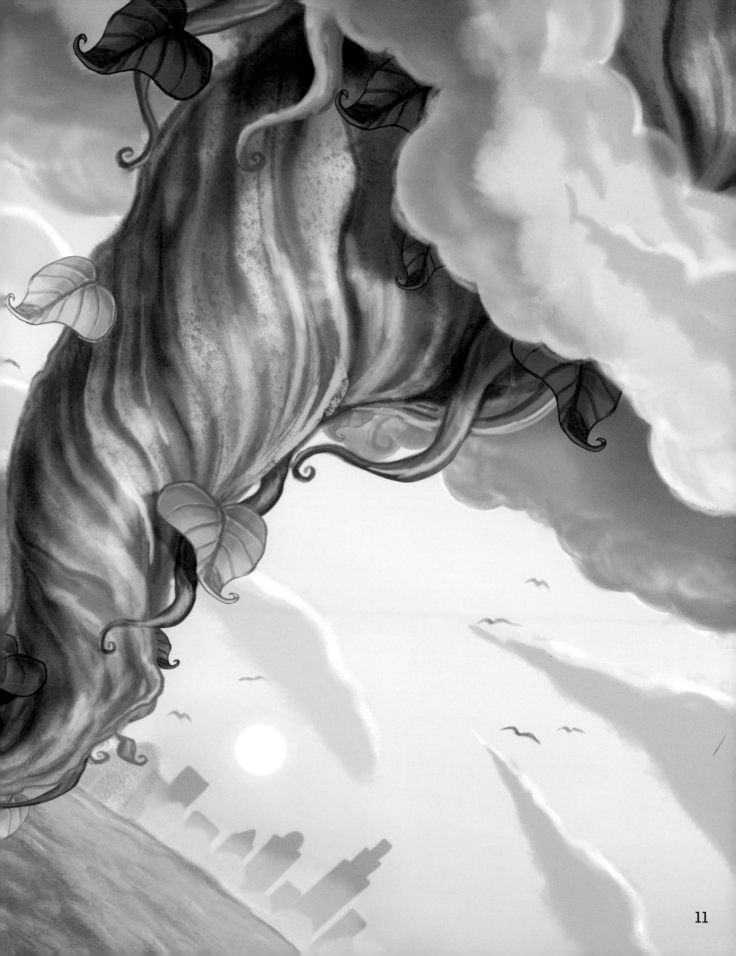

Jack gazed at the clouds. Maybe, just maybe, there was something to eat up there. He grabbed his gloves, gave his mom a hug, and started to climb.

He climbed pretty high. And then he climbed some more. After he climbed awhile, he, of course, did some additional climbing. Jack's house down below looked like a tiny speck.

"If I let go right now," he said, "gravity would pull me down. Fast. And that would hurt."

"Hey!" a voice boomed above Jack's head. "What are you doing, little guy?"

Jack froze.

"You look hungry, kid," the voice continued. "Come on up. I'll fix you a sandwich."

Jack had no idea whose voice it was. *But I am pretty hungry*, he thought. *How can I say no to a sandwich?*

So, with a loudly growling stomach, Jack climbed to the top of the beanstalk.

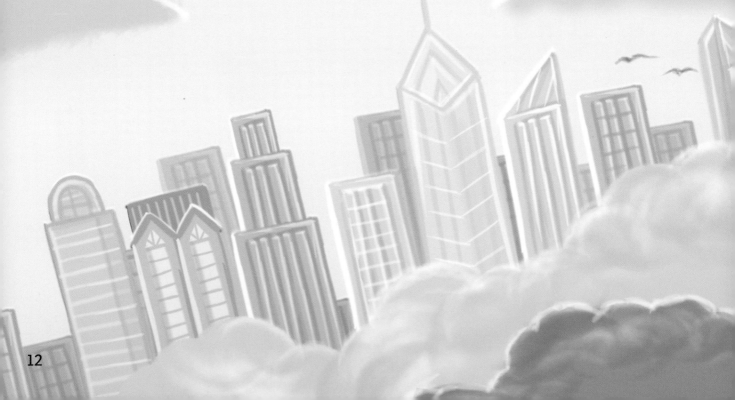

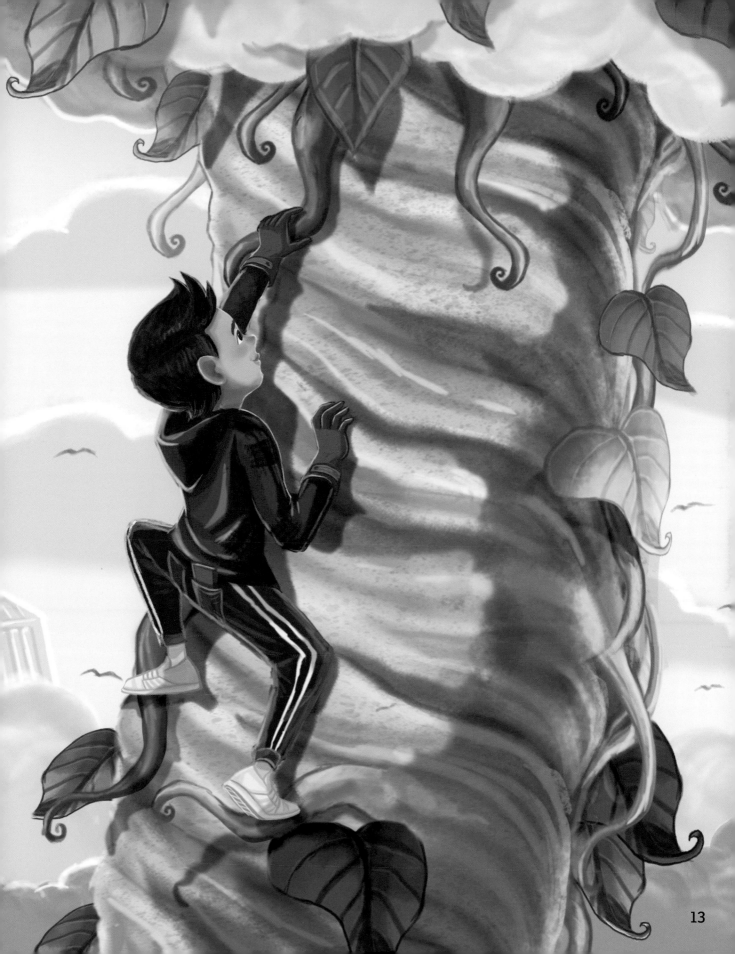

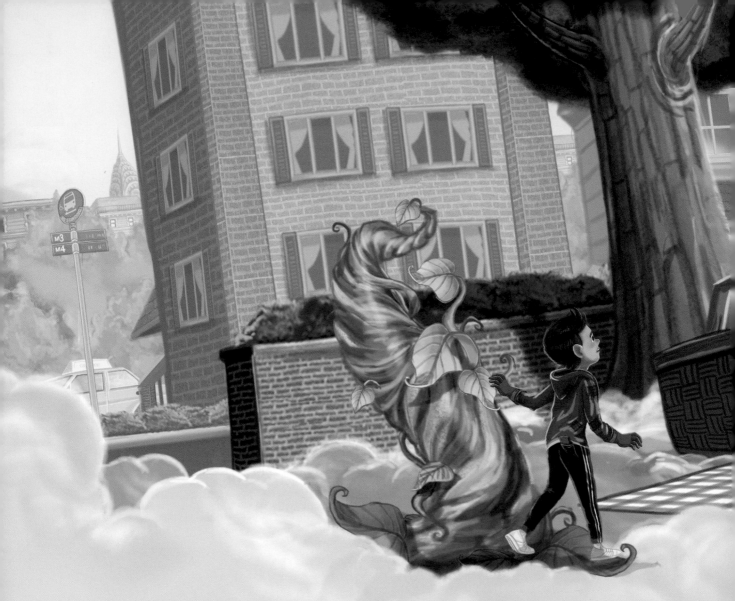

Everything above the clouds was big. Really big. Especially
the man sitting beside the beanstalk.

"Hey, kid," the giant boomed. "I'm Dennis."

"I'm Jack," Jack said.

"Please, enjoy this sandwich!" Dennis said. "It's going to stay
at rest until you eat it."

Jack raised an eyebrow. "Um . . . a sandwich at rest?" he asked.

"It's all about inertia," Dennis said. "Newton's First Law of
Motion says that objects will stay at rest (or in motion) until acted
upon by a force. The 'force' in this case is you!"

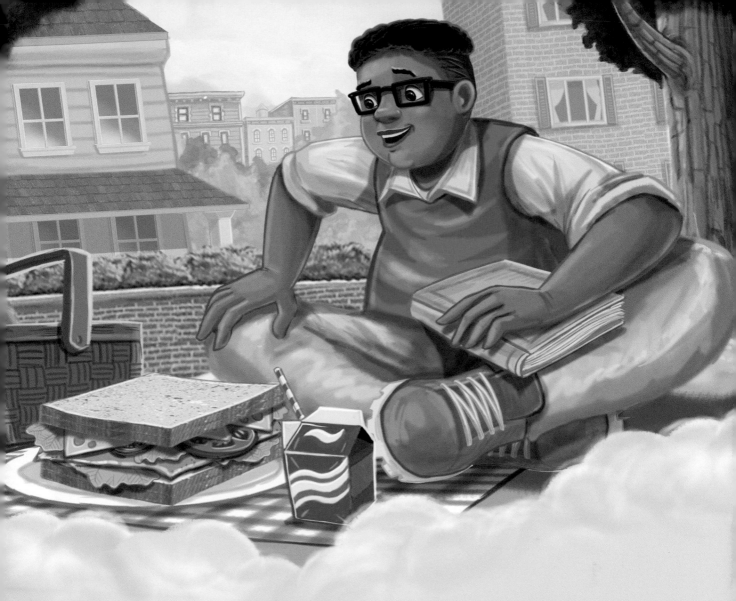

"Who's Norton?" Jack asked.

"*Newton.* Sir Isaac *Newton*," Dennis said. "He studied how objects move. Newton used his discoveries to create the Three Laws of Motion."

"So if I eat some of this delicious-looking sandwich, I'll disrupt its rest?" Jack asked.

"That's right," Dennis said.

"Well, then let's wake it up!" Jack said, tearing off a fistful of bread.

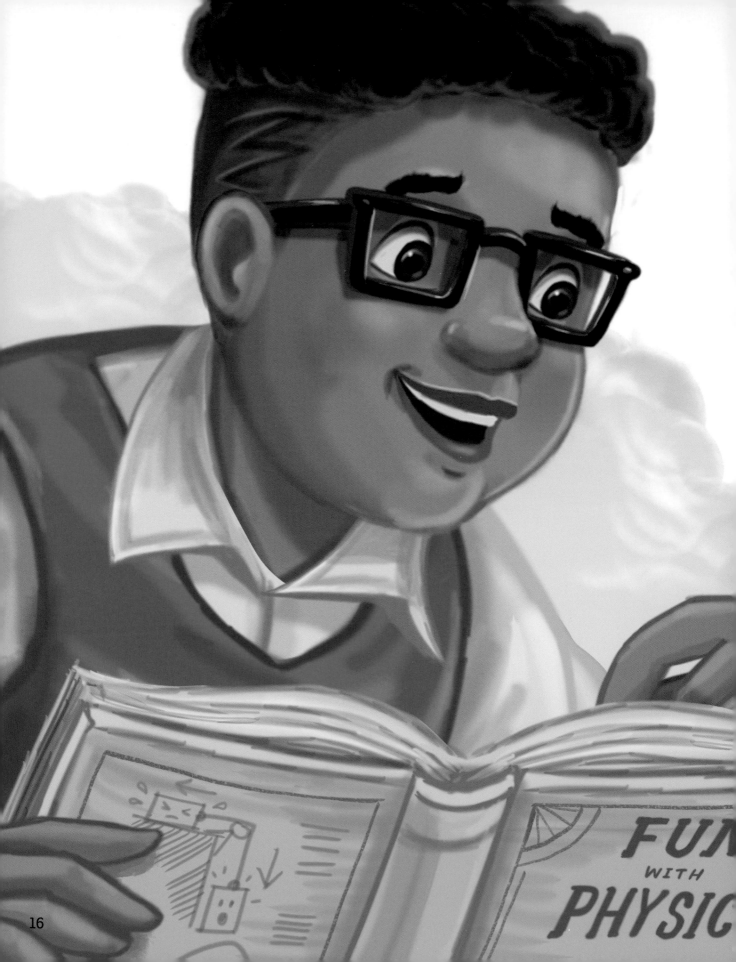

In surprisingly little time, Jack ate a big chunk of the sandwich. "So, Dennis," he asked, "are you a chef?"

"No," the giant said. "I'm studying to be a science teacher. I like figuring out how stuff works."

Jack pointed at the beanstalk. "That thing grew overnight from four magic beans," he said. "It's impossible to move. I tried."

"That's Newton's Second Law of Motion," Dennis said. He showed Jack a page from the physics book in his lap. "An object's speed can change based on its mass and the forces acting upon it."

"The beanstalk didn't move at *all* when I pushed on it," Jack said.

"Right, that's because the beanstalk has a much greater mass compared to you, little guy," Dennis said. "The more mass an object has, the more force is needed to move it. Now, if *I* tried . . ."

Dennis reached over and gave the huge beanstalk a tap. It wobbled.

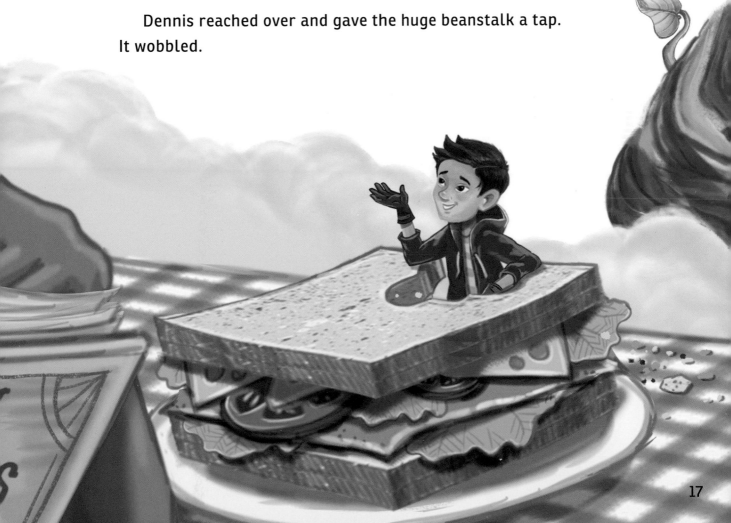

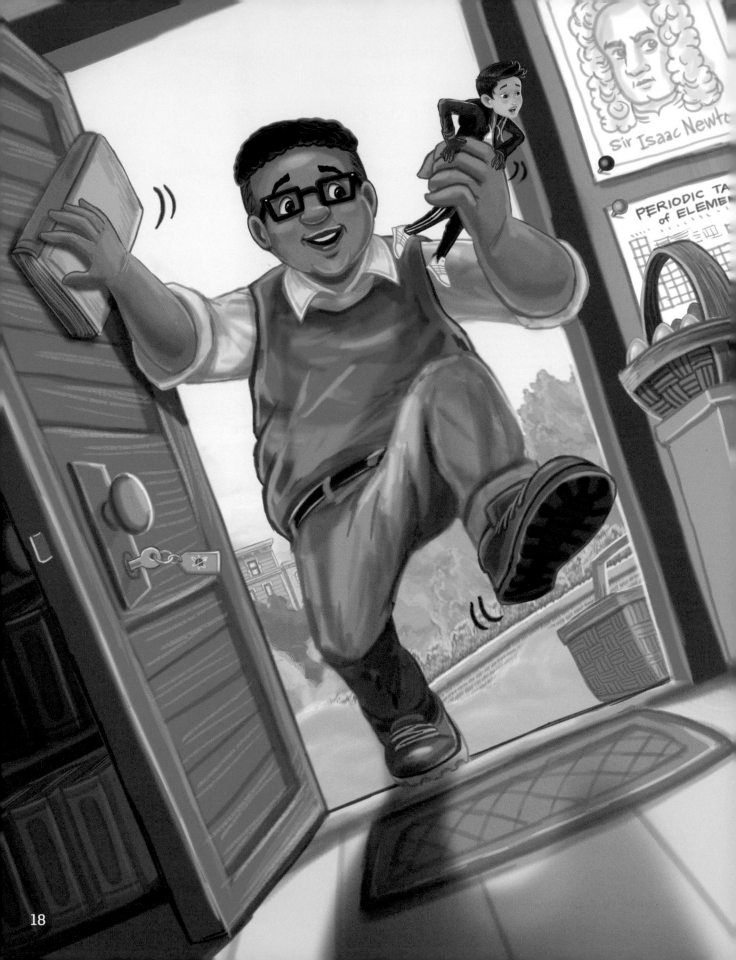

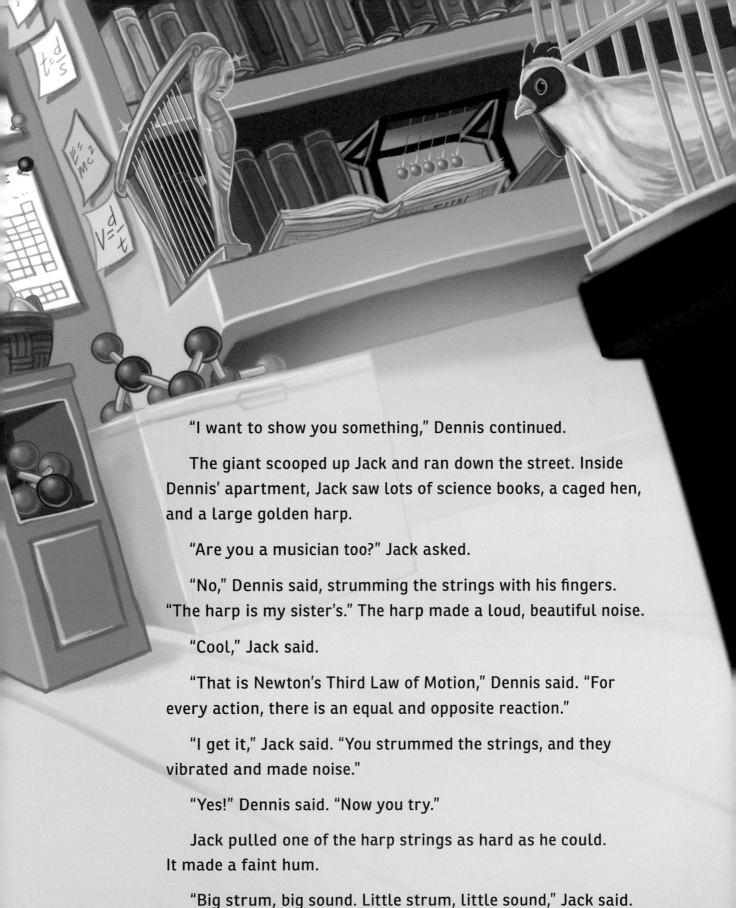

"I want to show you something," Dennis continued.

The giant scooped up Jack and ran down the street. Inside Dennis' apartment, Jack saw lots of science books, a caged hen, and a large golden harp.

"Are you a musician too?" Jack asked.

"No," Dennis said, strumming the strings with his fingers. "The harp is my sister's." The harp made a loud, beautiful noise.

"Cool," Jack said.

"That is Newton's Third Law of Motion," Dennis said. "For every action, there is an equal and opposite reaction."

"I get it," Jack said. "You strummed the strings, and they vibrated and made noise."

"Yes!" Dennis said. "Now you try."

Jack pulled one of the harp strings as hard as he could. It made a faint hum.

"Big strum, big sound. Little strum, little sound," Jack said.

Dennis' stomach rumbled and made the kitchen table shake. "You know, Jack," he said with a smile, "it's been a long time since I had a human for lunch."

"Um . . . what do you mean?" Jack asked.

"I mean, it's been a long time since I had company for lunch. It's nice," the giant explained, his stomach rumbling again.

"Oh," Jack said. "So how about a sandwich?"

"I'd love an omelet," Dennis said. "But my hen lays only golden eggs now. Sadly, you can't cook those."

Dennis picked up an egg and tossed it—**THUNK!**—in a basket nearly filled with other golden eggs.

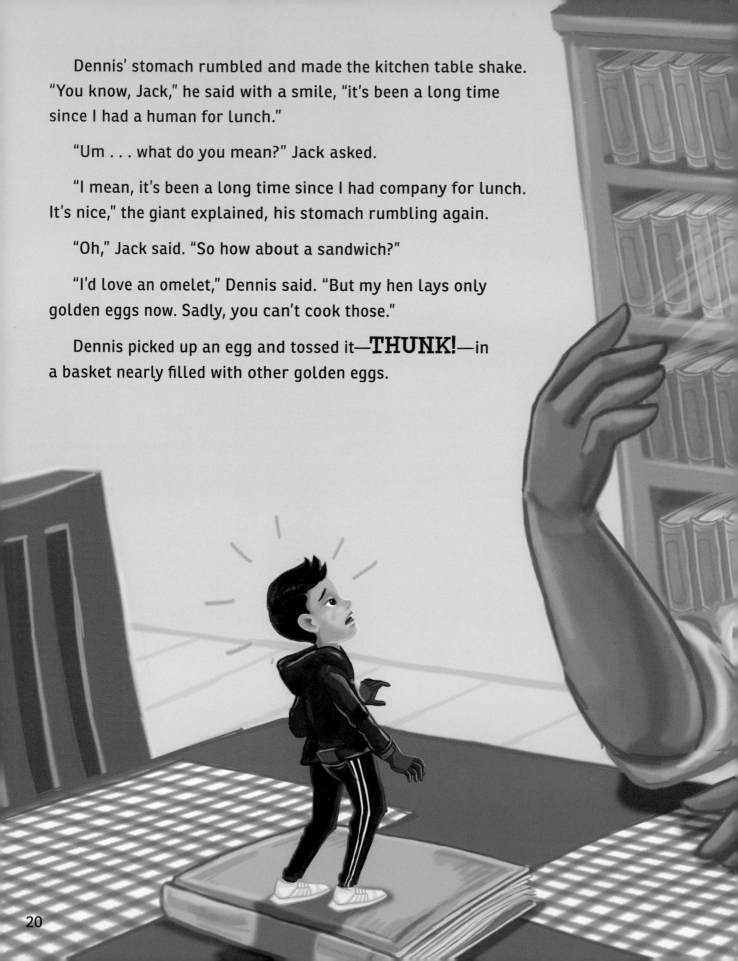

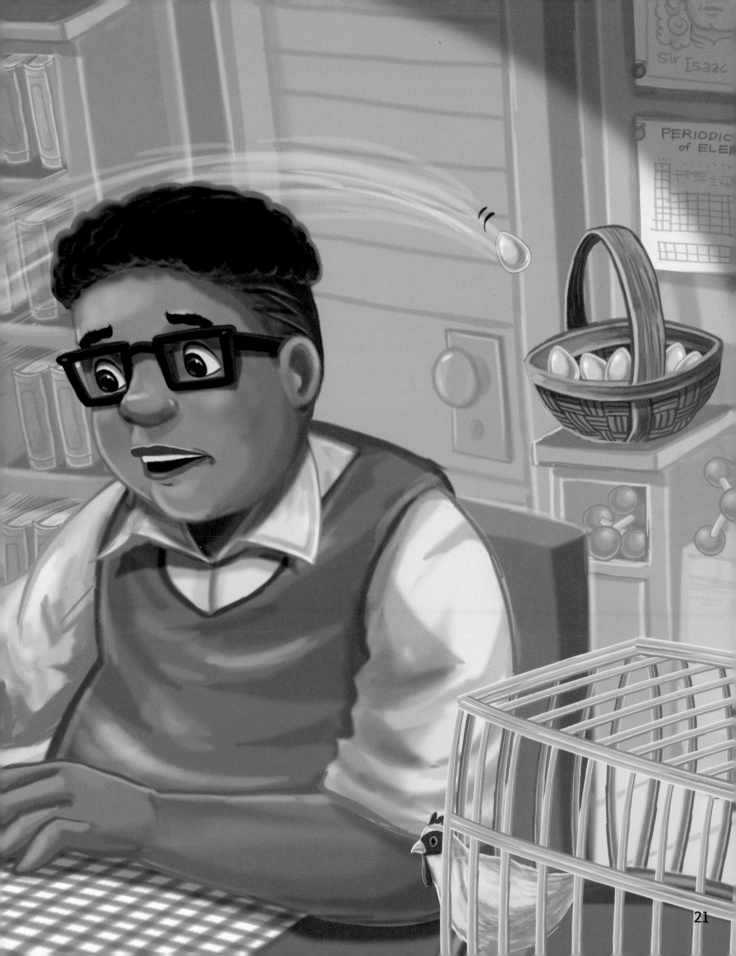

21

Jack didn't like the way Dennis was looking at him. If the giant's stomach growled once more, Jack needed to get out of the apartment—fast.

"Yeah," Jack said, "I hear ya. Golden eggs aren't helpful when you're hungry."

"Right," Dennis said. "I like omelets with mushrooms and Colby-Jack cheese."

"*Jack* cheese?!" Jack exclaimed. "That's it! I have to go!"

Quick as a flash, Jack jumped off the kitchen table and ran to the door.

"Wait! Where are you going?" Dennis asked.

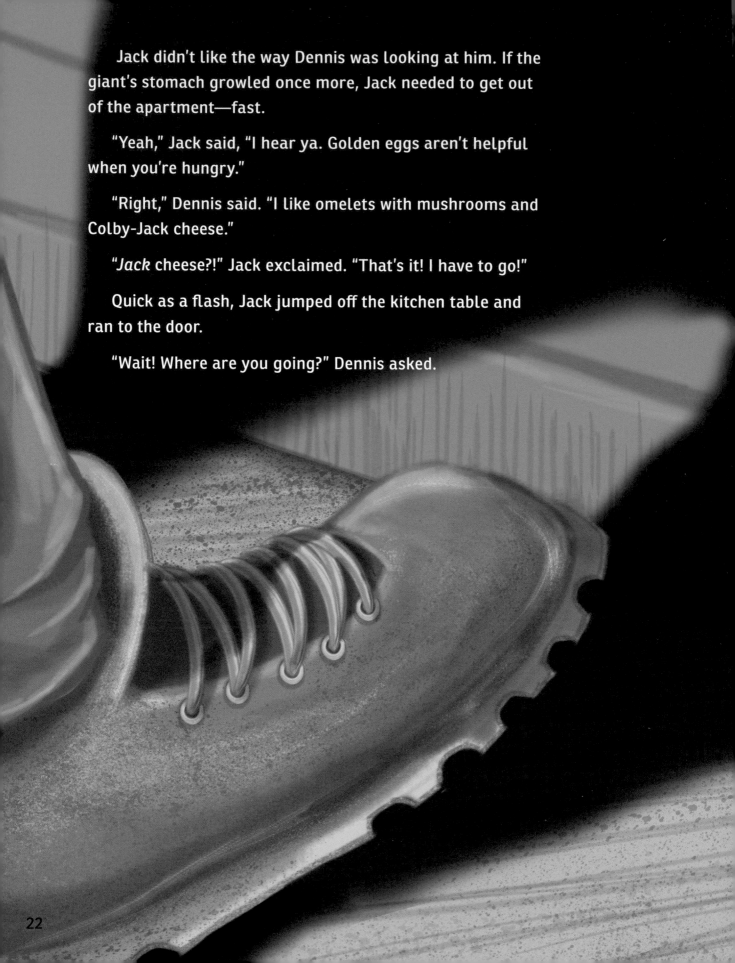

Jack pushed and pushed, but the door didn't budge. *Oh no,* he thought. *Not another one of Newton's Laws of Motion!*

"Fee, Fi, Fo, *Full*!" Dennis sang, walking up behind him. "This door opens with a *pull*!"

The giant pulled open the door, and Jack scrambled out.

"Hey, wait! What's your hurry, Jack? You forgot your—" Dennis shouted.

"Newton should have a *Fourth* Law of Motion," Jack cried, running as fast as he could. "Anyone chased by a hungry giant will move *really* fast!"

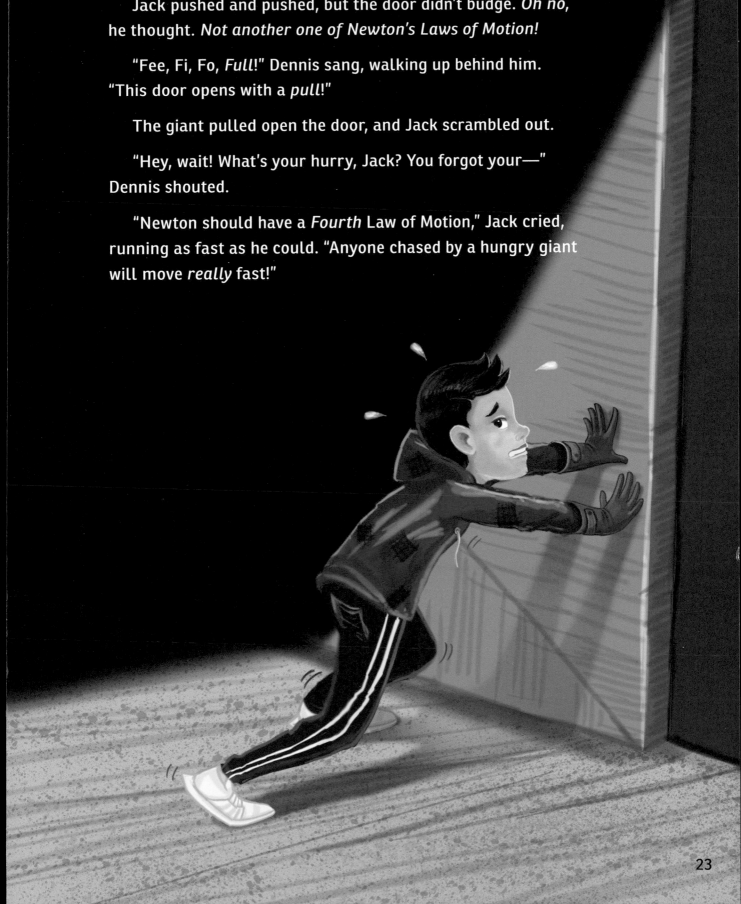

When Jack reached the beanstalk, he tightened his gloves and started sliding down. The giant followed.

"Gloves are a good idea, little guy," Dennis said. "They provide friction. Friction is what happens when the surface of one object meets another."

"How do you *know* all this stuff?" Jack cried.

"Friction can help slow you down," Dennis said. "It works in the opposite direction of motion. Please slow down so I can—"

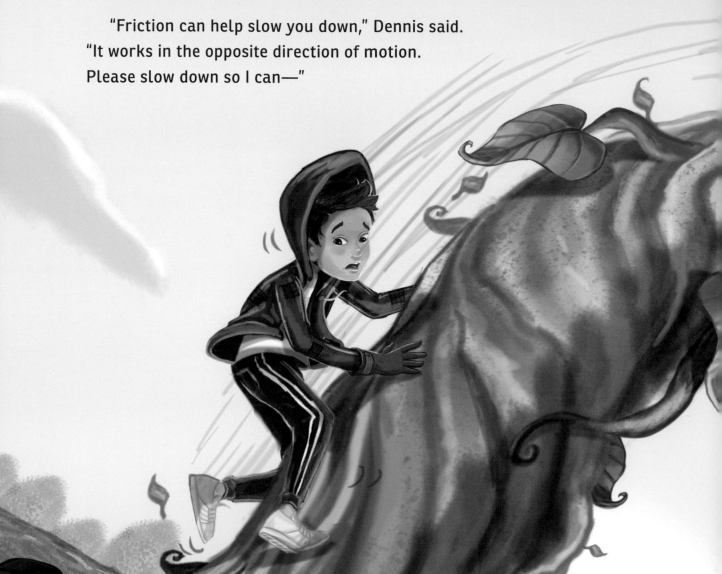

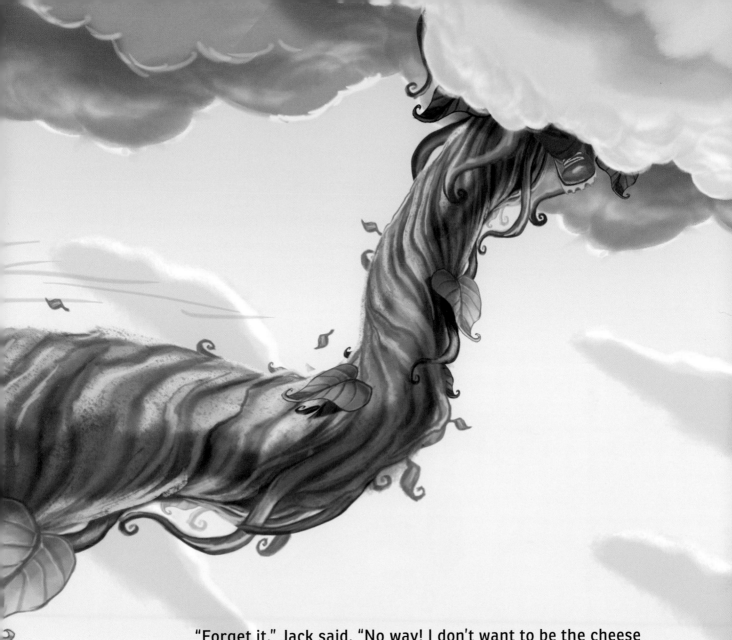

"Forget it," Jack said. "No way! I don't want to be the cheese in your omelet!"

Jack continued to slide toward home. The whole beanstalk shook as Dennis climbed down after him.

When Jack reached the ground, he yelled toward the house. "Mom! Get an ax! There's a giant coming down the beanstalk after me!"

A moment later, Mom ran out and tossed him an ax.

"Wait, Jack!" Dennis shouted from above.

Jack started to chop. He chopped a lot. And then he chopped some more. After a countless number of chops, he, of course, did some additional chopping.

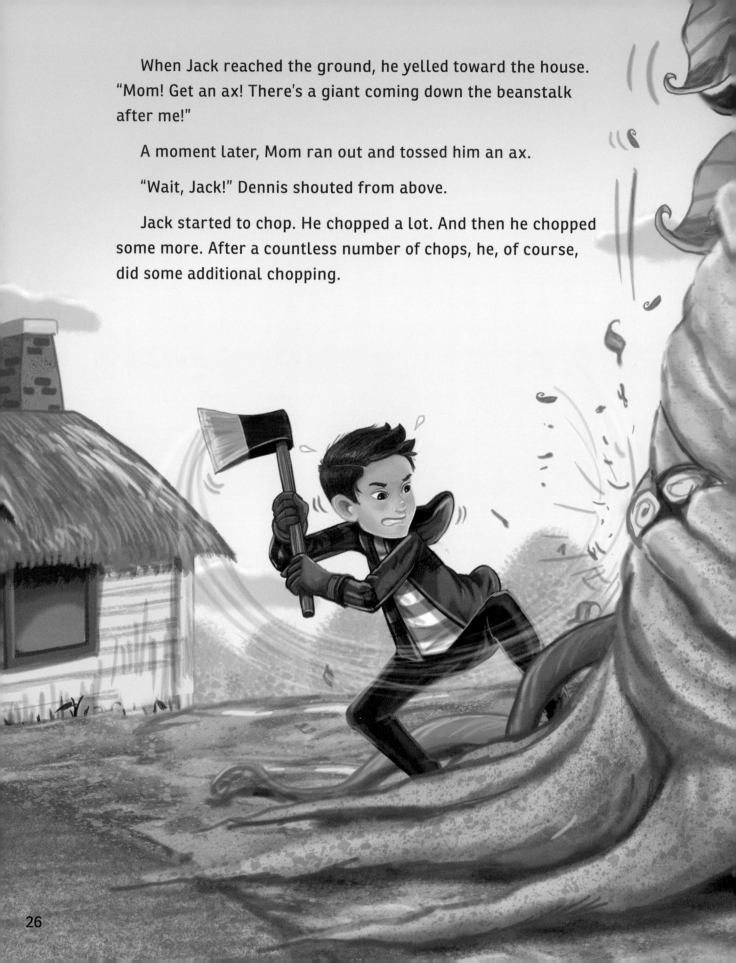

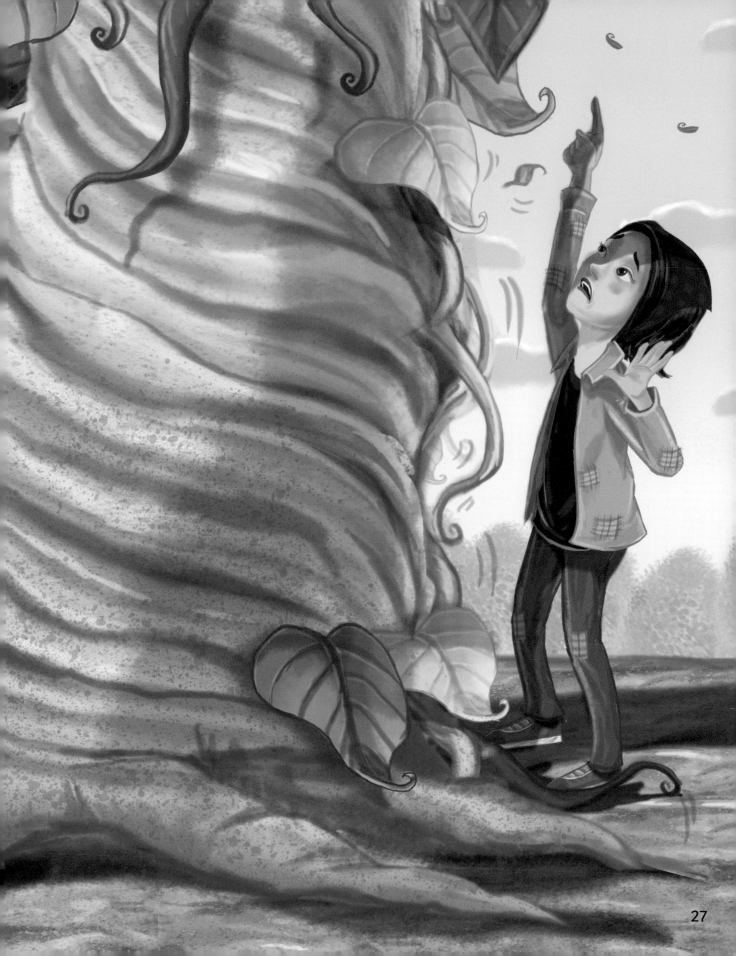

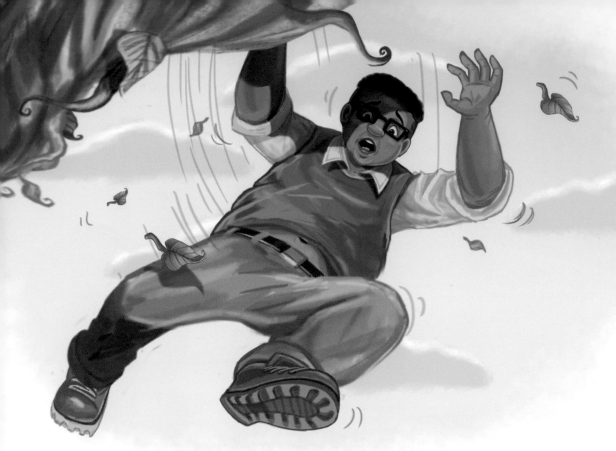

The beanstalk tipped, then toppled over.

Dennis landed. **BOOM!** Nearby houses collapsed.
A lake spilled into a valley. Somewhere a baby cried.

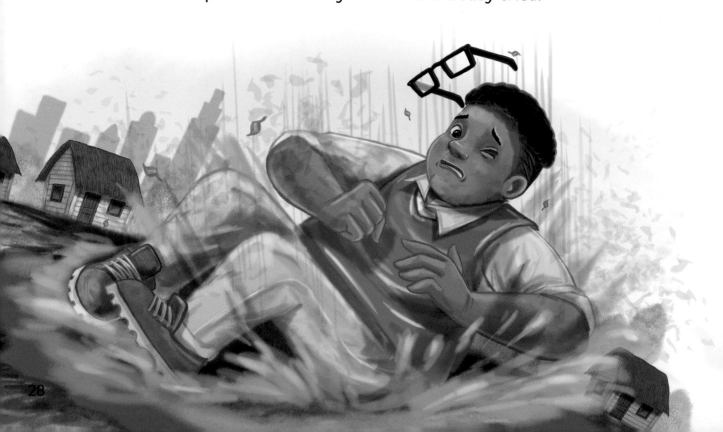

"Wow! What a drop! Thank goodness my shirt was loose and slowed down my fall," Dennis said. "It created drag, which acted in the opposite direction of motion—kind of like a parachute."

Jack sighed. "Yes, thank goodness," he said. "Well, go ahead and eat me. Get it over with. You wanted to eat me, right? That's why you were chasing me."

"No!" Dennis said. "You dropped your wallet at my apartment. Here."

Jack sheepishly took the wallet from the giant's hand. "Oh," he said in a very, very small voice.

Dennis smiled and asked, "What's for lunch, little guy?"

And so, stuck with a giant mouth to feed, Jack and Mom lived hungrily ever after. However, they did learn a lot about science.

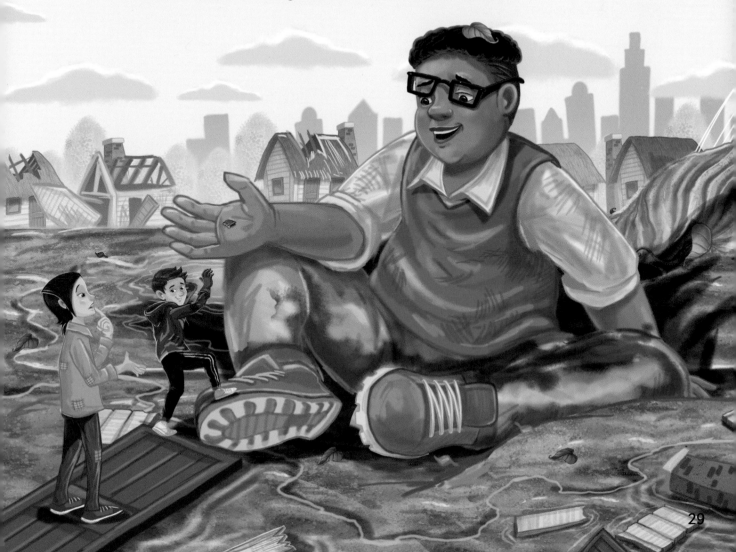

Glossary

drag—the force created when air strikes a moving object; drag slows down moving objects

force—a push or a pull

friction—a force created when two objects rub together; friction slows down moving objects

gravity—a force that pulls objects with mass together

inertia—a property of matter that makes objects resist changes in motion

law—a statement in science about what always happens when certain events take place

mass—the amount of material in an object

motion—movement

physics—the science that deals with matter and energy; physics includes the study of light, heat, sound, electricity, motion, and force

vibrate—to move back and forth quickly

Critical Thinking Questions

1. A force is a push or a pull. Give at least three examples from this story of a force in action.

2. Explain Newton's First Law of Motion using an object from your backpack.

3. Which would be harder for you: to push a baby stroller or a full-size car? Why? Use Newton's Second Law of Motion to explain your answer.

Read More

Barnham, Kay. *Isaac Newton.* Science Biographies. Chicago: Raintree, 2014.

Troupe, Thomas Kingsley. *Are Bowling Balls Bullies?: Learning About Forces and Motion with the Garbage Gang.* The Garbage Gang's Super Science Questions. North Mankato, Minn.: Picture Window Books, a Capstone imprint, 2016.

Winterberg, Jenna. *Balanced and Unbalanced Forces.* Huntington Beach, Calif.: Teacher Created Materials, 2015.

Internet Sites

Use FactHound to find Internet sites related to this book.

Visit *www.facthound.com*

Just type in 9781515828945 and go.

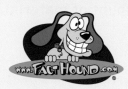

Look for all the books in the series!

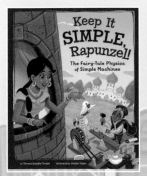
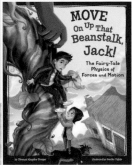
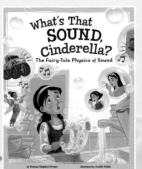
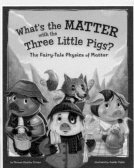

Index

Special thanks to our adviser, Darsa Donelan, Professor of Physics,
Gustavus Adolphus College, Saint Peter, Minnesota, for her expertise.

Editor: Jill Kalz
Designer: Lori Bye
Premedia Specialist: Tori Abraham
The illustrations in this book were created digitally.

Picture Window Books
1710 Roe Crest Drive
North Mankato, MN 56003
www.mycapstone.com

Library of Congress Cataloging-in-Publication data is available on the Library of Congress website.
ISBN 978-1-5158-2894-5 (library binding)
ISBN 978-1-5158-2898-3 (paperback)
ISBN 978-1-5158-2902-7 (eBook PDF)
Summary: When times are tough, you pull yourself up and push yourself to the top . . . of a beanstalk . . .
where you might get schooled in forces and motion by a STEM-loving giant named Dennis. At least that's
what happens to Jack in this delicious twist on a classic fairy tale.

Printed and bound in the United States of America.
042019   000075

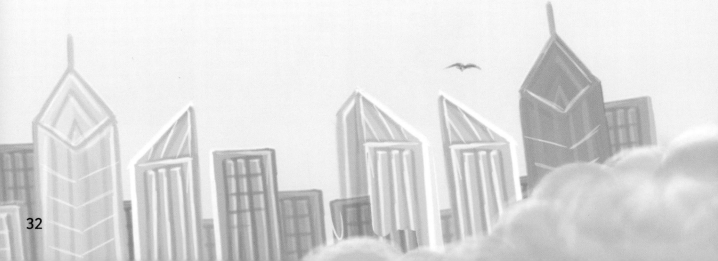